D0612742

Kenneth's Complete Book on Hair

Kenneth's Complete Book on Hair

Edited by Joan Rattner Heilman

Illustrations by Cornelia Smith

Doubleday & Company, Inc., Garden City, N.Y.

ISBN: 0-385-03299-4
Library of Congress Catalog Card Number 72-76167

Printed in the United States of America
9 8 7 6 5 4 3 2

CONTENTS

Kenneth's Complete Book on Hair

Chapter 1

A LITTLE ABOUT ME

Mine isn't an overnight success story. I've been at this business of hairdressing for almost twenty-five years. I think my success comes from the fact that I've never been involved with any one specific look in hair. Though I know I've been credited with creating the Bouffant hairdo, I don't think I invented it or that anybody else did. It was merely an evolution of a style. The fact is, I've never been known for up-to-the-minute styles, but rather for up-to-the-minute clients. By that I mean that real hair fashion comes from what women will wear on their heads—*they* are the final authorities. Most of my hairdos are really rather classic. But there must be something I do that's right because I have a very large regular clientele—some of them the most famous women in the world, some of them the richest women in the world; the rest, career girls, suburban housewives, teen-agers, society women. Some women come to me three times a week. Some come only twice a year. Some come every six weeks for a haircut. And I have many transient clients, people who visit New York once a year and want to have a marvelous time. Part of their trip is a trip to Kenneth's.

I've been asked, how come it's you? Why have you become one of the biggest names in hairdressing? I could give you a lot of stories about hard work and diligence, luck and all the rest. But there's more to it. My success is really a reflection of what's happened to hair in the last fifteen years, of being in the right place at the right time. Up until the mid-'50s, hair was not important. Flattering line or shape was achieved with hats. But with the advent of the Italian cut and the roller set, hair was in. And me with it. Hair became *the* most important fashion accessory.

And I've had an enormous amount of publicity. I can't deny the fact that having one of my regular clients go to the White House did have an enormous effect on the name Kenneth getting national exposure. Or the fact that I've been known as the hairdresser of celebrities like Marilyn Monroe, Lauren Bacall and Judy Garland. When I worked with Marilyn Monroe, my picture appeared in newspapers across the country. When Judy Garland made her sensational personal appearances, I traveled with her and my name was always mentioned as her hairdresser who was backstage.

Then, too, I was always willing to take time out of the salon, to give up substantial income, to spend a day or a week in a photographer's studio for the magazines. When I was first starting out at a big New York salon, I was bottom man on the totem pole, so I got all the discount customers—former employees of the salon, fashion people, assistant beauty editors. Nobody else wanted them because these were the "freebies." They would ask me to work on magazine and newspaper stories, setting hair for photography, and nobody else wanted that because there were no tips. But I enjoyed it and I became a better hairdresser on those stories—I got a chance to invent, to be creative. And I found myself with a fantastic clientele, a strangely powerful group of customers. The assistant beauty editors had become the beauty editors.

I always volunteered to go to the homes of customers and comb their hair before a major social function—and my name became known that way, too.

I've lasted longer than most hairdressers, I think, because I'm pliable. I enjoy change. It's easy to find a method or a look or a line which is temporarily unique to you. And it's easy to fall into the trap of sticking to it. You can ride a long time with it, but it doesn't last. You have to evolve your ideas and change them as you go. I try to talk women out of something I don't think they'd be happy with, even though it may be the "fashion" of the moment.

If I had to describe my "look," I'd say it was an unfettered, uncluttered, very real, very soft look. Even when, during a certain period, hairdos were more elaborate, perhaps using two or three hairpieces, mine always looked a little "undone." If a girl wore her hair in an upsweep, it looked like she'd managed to get it up there herself with just one hairpin. If you found that hairpin, it would all come tumbling down. I don't want to get involved with, and never have, the hairdo that's concrete. I've got to be right, too, at least for myself. If I had fallen into the trap of giving the customer what she *thinks* she wants—pastry-chef sculptures that you can't run your fingers through without breaking a fingernail—nobody would have heard of me and I wouldn't be writing this book.

I don't mean this as an ego trip, but I am basically a craftsman. I care very much about the kind of work I do. I want a customer to look good when she says her hair was cut by me. The important thing is that by the time a woman leaves me she feels she's prettier, more individual; that whatever it is she was looking for, I've accomplished it. Most people think this is a frothy business. I don't. I think it's a service business. Women come to Kenneth—this isn't, I hope, as vain as it sounds—because they think Kenneth can do something for them. You have to feel what people expect you to be, and then be it.

All the publicity in the world, no matter how many times your name is in the newspapers or pictures of your hair styles are in the magazines, really doesn't make you as well-known as a happy client, a woman who looks at herself when you're finished with her hair, and likes what she sees. I've received more publicity from women asking my clients, when they've seen them at a party or on the street, "Who did your hair?" than I have from anything else.

I never had any intention of becoming a hairdresser. I'd never known any and, as far as I can remember, I'd been in a beauty parlor only once when my mother had to take me along because she didn't have a baby sitter. My mother used to have her hair bleached and permanented and once she came home with all her hair broken off because she'd had a permanent on top of a bleach. But beyond these things, I don't remember even being curious about hair.

My hometown is Syracuse, New York, where I was born in 1927. I was the eldest of five children; the others were girls. It was a completely female world because my parents were divorced when I was twelve. I started working after school and summers then, and I had all kinds of jobs from dishwasher in the railroad-station restaurant to coffee boy while the trains were in the station. I ran an elevator in the tallest building in Syracuse and sold shoes in Grant's basement. I was a stockroom boy in a ball-bearings factory and sold beer in the baseball park.

When I was seventeen, just out of high school, I enlisted in the Navy, not because I was interested in going to sea but because it seemed more attractive than the infantry. I loathed military life. After boot camp, they decided somehow I'd be good material for the medical corps. I wasn't. Sticking a needle into somebody was a trauma. I was sent to watch an autopsy and had to be carried out. I was made a medical corpsman on a paraplegic ward, but I found it so depressing that I begged to be taken off. So I went to the officers' ward.

Two things happened the first day. First I was asked to give an enema to a very well-known silent screen star, who was then an admiral's aide. He threw a vase of flowers at me so I guess I didn't do my job too well. Then, I was asked to wax the floors with a waxing machine. Nobody took the time to show me how to control the thing, and it got away from me and crashed right through the wall of the building. The medical corps had a winner in me.

They realized this eventually, and I sold war bonds for a while, then took medical histories in a naval discharge center. Eventually I went through the discharge line myself.

Once out, I had to make a decision. What was I going to do now? I had a high-school education, pretty good marks, and not much money. I'd decided I wanted to be a psychiatrist but that wasn't feasible. I had to make money and help out at home.

I'd read an ad somewhere which said that the hairdresser's streets were paved with gold and it only took six months to learn how to be one. I wrote to *Vogue* magazine and asked the editors to recommend a school. I received a nice letter with a list of schools in

New York. I chose the smallest one, started out in New York and finished up in Syracuse.

I remember learning how to give permanents. The machineless waves were just coming in, but we learned how to do both machine and machineless. A friend of mine sent his mother in for a permanent one day and she wanted the old-fashioned kind. I got her all hooked up, which scared me to death as anything mechanical still does—I wince when I turn on the blender or plug in a lamp—turned on the machine and walked away. After a few minutes, I glanced over at her and saw a curl of smoke rising from the machine. I yelled for the teacher and ran over. All the woman had done was light a cigarette, but I was absolutely terrorized by the thought that her hair was being fried.

Toward the end of the school term, I got a part-time job at a small beauty salon during the Christmas rush. The first night, I arrived about six. At seven they gave me my first client, a middle-aged woman with shoulder-length hair. As I was about to wash her hair, she said, "My hair tangles very easily. I always use a vinegar rinse." I went back to the supply room but I couldn't find any vinegar. I did find a bottle which looked like a good thing and I poured a cup of it over her hair. I set her hair and I put her under the dryer.

When she was dry, I brought her back to the booth. Whatever I'd used had set her hair so stiff that I couldn't get the hairpins out. It was like plaster. The curls wouldn't move and I had to pull each one out and rub it between my fingers. All her hair would do was stand straight out in weird stiff strands. I couldn't even bend it.

She left and I left and I never went back there.

After I got out of school, I went to work in a little beauty parlor across the street from the Greyhound Bus station in Syracuse. It was a three-booth shop and I made $30 a week and a commission after I'd doubled my salary, plus tips. I worked very hard, thirteen or fourteen hours a day, six days a week. It was a very inexpensive beauty parlor but in six months, we became *the* shop in town. We raised the prices.

After two years, I decided to leave Syracuse and live in New

York. I was afraid to come here, though, so when a friend was going to Miami for the winter, I went along. I barely survived there.

In June of 1950, I arrived in New York with eight dollars and moved in with a friend from Syracuse who was living in a tiny apartment on the lower East Side. I wanted to work at Helena Rubinstein's which was the salon getting all the publicity at that time, but I was afraid to go there, so I went to Elizabeth Arden instead. I had never seen such a grand place. They gave me a model to work on. I did her hair and then everyone looked at my work and the man in charge said, "Well, it looks nice. Yes, we have a job for you—in our shop in Lexington, Kentucky."

I was so angry I marched right down the street to Rubinstein and asked for a tryout. They gave me the telephone operator who had wavy gray hair. I felt I knew the Rubinstein look and I copied it as closely as I could. All right, they'd try me out for two weeks at $50 a week. I was deliriously happy; I was exactly where I wanted to be.

The first day I worked there, I did two permanent waves. The first client gave me a five-dollar tip and the second one gave me a twenty-dollar tip. It was an auspicious beginning because I was used to twenty-five cents. Of course, I didn't do that well every day.

I stayed at Rubinstein's until 1956. This was the time, at least the first few years, when I had the last booth and all the clients nobody else wanted. I went out occasionally and worked on magazine sittings, arranging the models' hair, and getting to know the editors. Only the salon received the credit in the magazines, however; my name never appeared and I promised myself that if I ever owned a salon the individual hairdresser would get the credit for any hairdos he created that were seen in print.

It was also the time when a young woman came into the salon for an appointment with another hairdresser, who was out sick that day. I was the only one free at the time and they gave her to me. She was the wife of the then-junior senator from Massachusetts—Mrs. John F. Kennedy. I remember her as a very pretty girl who had short hair that was rather curly and had a mind of its own. I suggested she let it grow a little longer so the weight of the hair would help to stretch out some of the curl. And I felt the proportions of longer hair would be better. From that time on, she sometimes came to me and sometimes to the other man.

We had been setting hair with pin curls but the Italian cut changed that because it required lift. Rollers were generally unavailable then, so I had a dozen of them made up for me out of plastic. Everyone in the salon thought I was crazy, but the rollers did the job, and soon I became known around town as someone who did hair a little bit differently. But I was still only one of the thirty or forty hairdressers in the salon.

One day in 1956, two models, clients of mine—Melissa Weston and Gillis McGill—suggested that I go for an interview with Lilly Daché who had opened a salon which wasn't getting off the ground. I went. Miss Daché offered me the job of style director of her salon and I took it.

Now my name appeared on everything I created for the newspapers and magazines. We became the most important salon in New York and had many famous clients from all over the world.

Mrs. Kennedy was one of my clients who followed me to Daché, and when she went to the White House, I was often asked to go down to Washington to do her hair before most of the important social functions—including the inauguration. Obviously, it wasn't practical for me to be her only hairdresser at such a distance, so we asked a Washington hairdresser to train to take over. We wanted him to see what I did with her hair. When he found out that he occasionally might have to be at the White House at seven-thirty in the morning, he didn't want the job. He turned it down. I was amazed—I would have been there at 3 A.M. if necessary. Maybe I was terribly naive, but it was always a tremendous thrill for me to go through the White House gates—the last time I did was the day before the President was assassinated.

While I was at Daché, my day began about eight or nine in the morning and often didn't end until about ten at night. The salon wasn't open then, of course, but I'd often comb hair in the clients' homes before a big event. I'd be exhausted by the time I'd get home to my apartment but I loved it.

Whether this is what many other people would want is, of course, questionable. I have subjugated my personal life to my business. I like doing what I do and it has never bothered me to work so hard or so long. Other people often aren't fortunate enough to be able to make the choice—they marry early, have children, or have a life outside of their work that is more important to them. Certainly I can understand that. But the way I lived suited me.

And it was exciting. Soon after I arrived at Daché, I accompanied the beauty editor of *Glamour* magazine and a photographer on a trip to several exotic countries of the Near and Far East. The idea was to photograph royalty in these countries and bring a sense of Eastern magic to a Christmas issue. Unfortunately, whoever had been charged with setting up the arrangements had goofed and everywhere we went, we were a complete surprise to the palace.

Our first stop was Morocco where we were to photograph the sister of King Hassan. When we arrived in Rabat and telephoned the palace, we discovered they'd never heard of us. We explained our mission and then for two days we waited for word. Finally we were asked to appear at the palace at nine o'clock that night. We were picked up at the hotel, taken to the palace, through the guards, through a courtyard, arriving at a side entrance. As we stepped into the doorway, all the blazing lights of the palace went out. We stood frozen in a blackened reception room, waiting for something to happen. Finally someone appeared with a candle. We were escorted through a maze of rooms to a big hall and introduced to the princess whom we couldn't see very well. After conversation about our mission, she agreed to pose for the pictures and we chose a beautiful ceremonial robe with an enormous jeweled belt for her to wear.

Unfortunately, when we finally saw the princess in the light we discovered that, like many women in Morocco, she hennaed her hair. Because she hadn't expected us, she hadn't had her henna pack in quite some time. About two inches of her own dark hair showed, the rest was red.

We took the pictures and she was very kind to us, but we were never able to use them.

Leaving our hotel to catch the plane onward, I fell down an enormous flight of marble stairs, scattering my rollers and clips and hairpins in every direction. Getting on the plane, I cracked my head on the door. The whole thing was a disaster.

We flew to Amman in Jordan where we were to photograph King Hussein's new wife, Muna. She didn't expect us either. But in twenty-four hours we were asked to come to the palace for an interview and state why we were there. At the gates, we and the car were thoroughly searched, then we were taken to one of the king's aides. Finally we arrived at the king's quarters. He himself greeted us and seemed to understand our mission though I don't think we did at that moment. He took us inside, introduced us to his wife and left.

I trimmed her hair and set it. When it was dry, she went to her closet and picked out a pale blue-green dress to wear. We all went out on the terrace which overlooked the entire city. Below us were a row of guards with machine guns.

It was August and it was hot. Muna stood in a corner so Amman could be seen in the background. I went over to her to pin her hair on the side because it was blowing in the breeze, and as I did it, she slumped to the floor. She had fainted. I nearly fainted too. We started to lift her up to carry her in out of the sun when I said, "For heaven's sake, don't touch her!" I couldn't imagine what those men down there would do if they saw us with the limp body of the queen in our arms.

Again we didn't have a picture. Two days later, though, we went back and got one.

That's the way our trip went.

I think I've been very lucky to have had such extraordinary exposure to so many worlds. I've shared a small part of some great people's lives. I've been in some of the richest homes in the world, I've gone around the world three times for magazines, stayed in the most luxurious hotels, been entertained by people in very high places. And I've learned marvelous things that have enriched my life. But I've never become involved in the lives of my clients. I don't socialize with them. I had a brief fling at it. I was once invited to a dinner party by a client. After dinner, her husband stayed home and she and I went on to another party held on a huge yacht on the Hudson. The next day it was all over the papers: "Pickle Queen goes to Yacht Party with Hairdresser." I hated it and that was the end of that. That's not what life is all about, not for me anyway.

There's an old saying in the publicity field—it doesn't matter what they say about you as long as they spell your name right. I don't believe that. I care very much what they say and I'd rather not be mentioned at all except in a professional context. I have developed a life outside my work which doesn't involve my clients and that's the way it should be.

I feel the same way about my clients. I discourage gossip. I'm not particularly interested in other people's private lives. I have enough to worry about my own. And I don't like to tell private stories about my clients because their lives are really none of my business. Anyone who's involved in a personal service business can tell plenty of secrets. And everyone would love to hear them. Scandal is fun. But I won't be part of it. If the clients want to tell, fine. I simply will not. Some of the press used to get extremely irritated when I wouldn't tell in great detail what I knew about the then Mrs. Kennedy and her hair. But if you were my client, would you like me to tell something I'd overheard you say to or about your husband, or the way you speak to your children? I can't believe anybody who's lucid would want this.

So there will be many things left unsaid, because they won't help anyone have a better head of hair.

The only stories I've ever told have not been private information. Marilyn Monroe was one of my steady clients, and I did her hair until the time she died. The first time I met her she was finishing *Some Like It Hot* and was having problems with her hair which had been overbleached and, she felt, was too curly. Her secretary called me and asked me to come over to her apartment with my equipment. Of course, I was very excited by the whole idea. I took my bag of rollers and clips and I went. I waited very nervously in a white and beige foyer for about a half hour till Marilyn came in, in a white terrycloth robe and a big towel around her wet hair, just as nervous as I was. I was staggered by how beautiful she was just that way with no makeup and no hairdo.

I blunted the ends of her hair and gave it a bias setting to try to overcome some of her strong wave pattern, making it look almost straight but turned up at the ends all the way around. She put on her makeup—it took her about an hour to do it, and then wiped most of it off for a marvelous subtle effect—and then a nude-color beaded chiffon dress that looked almost glued on her. She looked terrific.

She was extremely shy and unsure of herself through this whole meeting. But I remember when she walked out later into a roomful of strangers, she suddenly became another woman, the woman we all saw in her pictures.

When *Some Like It Hot* had its world première in Chicago, I went with her to prepare her for her stage appearance of which she was terrified. I combed her hair out on the plane before we landed to confront a pushing, shoving, grabbing mob scene at the airport.

We piled into a car and headed for the theater—Marilyn, a publicity man and myself. When we approached the theater, the car was suddenly surrounded by thousands of screaming people trying to get near her. They climbed on the car, trying to get in, to get a look at her, to touch her. I locked the doors as the mob started to rock the car back and forth, side to side. Marilyn was near hysterics, and we were all terrified. We inched our way forward and finally got to the theater entrance in a state of near collapse.

I thought to myself, you'd have to be mad to want that kind of attention.

When the photographers crowded around after her appearance, Marilyn insisted that I be in the pictures too. Those pictures of Marilyn Monroe and Kenneth Battelle, formerly of Syracuse, were printed all over the world.

The last time I saw her was six weeks before she died, when she agreed to do a few pages for *Vogue*. I flew to California to do her hair. As she was posing for the last shot—lying on the floor with her hair spread out all around—I had to run for the airport to catch my plane. She asked me to kiss her good-by. I did, and I never saw her again. All of a sudden she was gone. I have always wished I'd recognized the depth of her loneliness—perhaps I could have been a better friend if I had.

I remember doing Lucille Ball's red hair one day. When she came to the top of the stairs in the salon, she asked, "Where's God?" which made everybody laugh, including me. She is probably one of the most delightful, relaxed people I've ever known. I decided to play a trick on her. After her hair had been cut and set and dried, I started combing it. I brushed it out, teased it very high and wild all over her head—it was in the days of the Bubble. Then I put down the brush and said very seriously, "Thank you very much. I hope you enjoy your hair." And I left the booth.

She just sat there and I hid in the lunchroom. Suddenly there was a shriek: "He's not *serious?*" At which point I went back, finished combing her hair and we had a good laugh.

One day a model-friend of mine came into the salon with one of the most extraordinary-looking people I'd ever seen. It was Kay Kendall. My friend knew her, had met her on the street, persuaded her not to go to the hairdresser with whom she had an appointment but to come to me. Kay had just arrived in New York from Hollywood where they'd made her hair that famous technicolor red. It was long and she was wearing it in a thick French twist.

After I gave her her new hair style, it became an overnight sensation—we had people lined up at the salon to get their hair done this way. I cut her long hair because so much of it was in bad condition and toned down the red as near as possible to her own natural brown. She was a very tall woman with a head almost too small for the rest of her body, so I couldn't make her hair too tight and tiny. It ended up about four or five inches long all over her head, set on small rollers, teased, and brushed up with tendrils in front of each ear.

She wore her hair that way from then on, came in regularly for a cut, bringing a bag of hamburgers for everybody because she thought we all should have a hot lunch.

Of course, as most people do, I'd always dreamed of having my own business. And in 1963, I opened my own salon. Having been a child of the depression and an avid movie-goer, I had a vision of a House of Beauty with masseuses and mud-pack rooms and chiffon drapes and a hundred doorways with mysteries behind each one. A completely impractical idea, but I wanted to come as close to it as I could.

I took an old five-story mansion on East 54th Street. It had been built in 1895 and was a private home until about 1920. I wanted to keep the sense of a private home and to have a luxurious comfort that would also be practical. I had seen the Brighton Pavilion in England not long before and I loved the sheer mad fantasy, the sense of humor and luxury of it. That was the effect I wanted in my salon.

I asked Billy Baldwin to do the decorating, and it worked out just the way I wanted it to. We used a lot of pattern on pattern, cotton-draped walls, wicker furniture, flowered carpeting, lacquer paint in brilliant colors. I avoided all the fake French dressing-room decor that so many salons have, stayed away from the aqua, baby blue and gold angels and that kind of thing. As a result, there is a wonderful sense of luxury and humor and permanence about the place.

We had some very funny reactions to it. Some people said it looked like a Chinese restaurant. Others said it looked like a bordello. All of which pleased me because nobody said it looked like a beauty salon.

At Daché, as director of the salon, I only cut hair. The sets and other work were done by other people. At my salon, I do the same. It started as a way to cope with large numbers of clients, to keep my hand in, to have some relationship with each client. And it was the beginning of what's going on in hairdressing today—it started the upgrading of the haircut as the basis of a hairstyle.

I now do what pleases me. I spend half a day in the salon. I make store appearances, do a lot of television and newspaper interviews, photographic sittings. We've taken a stab at the cosmetic business, sell a line of wigs. It's a very interesting life.

Chapter 2

MY PHILOSOPHY OF HAIR

My favorite look for hair is clean, shiny, bouncy, soft, free and healthy. It must have absolute reality, it must look natural. Hair is beautiful if you let it be hair. It's basically a beautiful fabric, a marvelous material which can be glorious if it's treated with respect. If it isn't—if it's forced to do something it wasn't meant to do—it's no longer hair, it's a mess.

Hair should *look* like hair. It should be comfortable, something you can take care of yourself after you've left the salon. This leaves out excessive teasing, hair that is lacquered into a stone, hair colors that are unbelievable. It leaves out hair that's been tormented and mistreated until it's a mass of dry straw. Women do terrible things, idiotic things, to their hair in the name of beauty. They get this once-beautiful fabric in awful shape and then they look for a magical solution. There isn't any.

Style isn't nearly so important as good health, good treatment and a good haircut, though I have to admit I'm always amazed by the number of women I see who have startlingly wrong hairdos for them. Your hair should be decorative, make you look pretty, but it should look like it's part of you and not a piece of sculpture—or a bird's nest—sitting on top of your head. Yet it must have line.

The important thing is the haircut. If you have a bad haircut, forget it. Your hair just won't do what it should. If you have a good one, it will look fine even when it's not set or when the set is several days old.

There are no miracles. There are lots of women who like to believe that there's somebody named Kenneth—or Pierre or Mary or Josephine—who will make them instantaneously beautiful with no responsibility of their own. There's no such thing. I like to think I can work miracles, but I really can't. People don't want to hear that but it's true. I can help, certainly, but the way you look is really a matter of caring, of paying attention to yourself. You can't have a Kenneth in your coat pocket. For example, you buy a beautiful wig. You are shown how to wear it, how to tuck your own hair under it. The first time you wear the wig, you remember. The second time, you're in a hurry and get it on all wrong, with ends of your own hair hanging out around the edges. A professional can only point the way. After that, you are on your own.

Your hair will do only what its texture will allow it to do. Few women want to learn, if they have baby-fine hair, that a simple chin-length blunt cut is best for them. They don't want to know it. But that's what it's all about. You must take the material you've got—your hair—and make the best you can out of it. It's different from your best friend's and it's different from your sister's. It has its own special individual qualities, and that's what you've got to work with.

Your hair texture determines how long your hairdo will "keep." Baby-fine hair won't hold a set very long; fine hair has a certain amount of "hold or body"; medium-textured hair has even more hold; and coarse hair has the most. The degree of curl or wave your hair has will also affect the lasting power of your set.

Never before at any time in recent history that I can remember have people had so much opportunity to look their own way as they have today. There is no real fashion in hair today. There's no real fashion in anything now. All that is dead. It's over, it's finished. No one dictates the mode the way it was done just a few years ago. There will always be tiny waves, small fads—kinky hair, bare feet, straight hair, long hair, shirts and ties—but fashion dictates, as they once were known, are finished.

Today's hairdo is tomorrow's throwaway. It's as instant as that. Everything changes constantly and immediately, hair included. It is a passing symbol.

Hairdressing as we have known it is over, too, I think. In the next ten years, the whole business is going to be completely transformed, and it's changing faster than many of us are willing to admit. Older women will continue to go to hairdressers for their semi-weekly or weekly shampoos and sets, but they will soon be very much in the minority. The younger people will go only for super cuts, scalp treatments, great coloring or other special things, and men and women will go to the same places to get their hair done, i.e., cut.

Perhaps the hair will be set in some way, or arranged by blowing it dry or drying it with heat lamps or letting it dry in place. Perhaps some rollers will be used, or pin curls, or a curling iron or even permanent waving. But everything will be based on the ability of the clients themselves to keep their hair looking good for weeks at a time between appointments.

I think the only hairdressers who will survive this change and the only clients who will really look good will be those who understand this trend. I don't think that this is necessarily bad, though it's surely not good for the hairdressing business as it is structured today.

Today you can elect to wear any style you want. You can wear short pants, long pants, curly hair, straight hair, hair pulled back in a bun, hair in a tangled mass of curls or in a crew cut, skirts to your ankles or to the bottom of your behind. You can be completely casual or completely formal. It is all there to choose from.

I think that's terrific, but I've found it terrifies most women. They don't like it! Unfortunately, they don't want the responsibility of deciding for themselves. They want to be told what to do, how to look. They feel they *must* fit into a certain mode of fashion, that they *have* to wear their hair in some particular way that's current at the moment.

One question I hear almost more than any other is "What is the new hairdo?" There are always styles that are especially popular, but I hope we are growing up and away from THE HAIRDO, with everyone wanting the same thing or a version of it. I wish people were really willing to be more individual. Wanting *the* hairdo, whether it's a freaky, revolutionary style or a long Shag, a page boy or the perfect "coif," is a search for identification. It's a way of fitting into a particular life style, of being safe, of being part of one's group. Probably the best thing, if you can do it, is to try not to wear a uniform on your head, but to do the best you can with your own hair, to try to be individual as well as pretty.

I personally try to fight conformity by giving each client what I think *she* looks good in, what works well with *her* hair and what she'll be comfortable with, a hair style she can cope with when she's left the salon. I like to think I never make anybody look like a freak. I like to think I make women look prettier.

Most distinctively beautiful women—the Duchess of Windsor, Jackie Onassis, Ali McGraw, Catherine Deneuve, Audrey Hepburn, Sophia Loren, Mrs. William Paley, Elizabeth Taylor, to name a few famous ones—have always defied "fashion" in hair styles, long before this age of freedom. They have each found a certain hair style for themselves, and have stayed with it, through all the changing currents. They've made fashion suit themselves and haven't followed every little mode that's come along. They have found a look of their own, a style of their own. And, with some minor changes over the years, they have stayed with a basic line which comes from a true knowledge of themselves. If they've always worn their hair long, they wouldn't think of cutting it off because "everyone's doing it." If they've always worn a chignon, or a soft wave or a French twist, they've still got it. They know how they look best. Consequently, they can be both beautiful and individual.

All of the women I know who are considered great beauties are not necessarily women born prettier than anyone else. Nor are they necessarily rich. They are women who have a positive approach to their looks. They have tried things that may have been disastrous but they've had the sense to realize that and quickly change it.

One outstanding example occurs to me. This was a client I had several years ago who is now considered internationally a great beauty. She has an enormous hooked nose. Before she came to me, she'd been told she must always wear bangs or hair around her face to help hide the size of her nose. I made her grow her hair long and put it straight back tight to her head in a small bun on the back. It was a deep but indefinite brown and I asked her to have it tinted brown-black. She did. She learned how to make up her eyes to the best advantage. She is now really spectacular.

Unfortunately, most of us don't have the desire or the courage to get out of the mainstream and to do what is really best for us. The younger people today have much more of that sense of what is best for them than the older ones—the over twenty-fives. And, hopefully, they will give individuality the good name it deserves.

Kids today have a wonderful look. They're healthy and vital and attractive in every sense. Some are dirty and untidy, of course, but those are in the minority. Most young people look great. Why? Because they're not locked into a rigid style. And I think they'll always be the same way. Today's twenty-year-olds, when they are thirty-five, are not going to look like today's thirty-fives. They're not going to do the same things to their hair.

Many young women now are trying to follow the "natural" route. They want to keep the kind of hair they were born with and work with that, rather than try to change it altogether as their mothers do.

The other day a sixteen-year-old girl came into my salon to see me. She came with her mother who is a regular client. She had very thick fine hair that was very, very curly, almost frizzy, rather like a big mattress on top of her head. And it was long, below her shoulders.

She said to me, "Could I have my hair slightly trimmed so it would be smoother?" I explained that no kind of trimming, or even cutting, was going to smooth her hair. I told her that perhaps a straightening would do the job.

She wouldn't consider that—because it was "unnatural." This was a complete changeabout from a few years ago when girls would do anything in the world to get straight hair.

I said, "Fine, then why don't you have it cut in a shape and wear it really natural. Wash it, towel-dry it, and push it into shape."

Well, maybe that was *too* natural.

We compromised on a very blunt haircut that left all the length, and I showed her how to wrap set the hair to get some of the curl out when she wanted to take the bother to do it. But, basically, she decided to live with her own hair.

I'm not for or against natural or unnatural. It all depends, as in all things in life, on a woman's ability to cope with what she's got. Some people enjoy hair that's got what other people would consider a problem, and they use it. Other people can't stand it, and so they try to change it. When they think of it as a problem and they come to me, I offer solutions. Then it's their decision what to do. Someone who's seventeen may well be happy with her very curly hair and use it in an advantageous way. After all, all her peers are doing the same thing. But it's hard for somebody who is, perhaps, forty-two and has always considered her curly hair excessive and even disfiguring, to think about letting it go natural now.

Beauty is not the most important thing in the world, by any means. But it is a way people remember us and it is a way of communicating. Today we are judged first by our façades. It may be sick, but that's the way it is. People are more attracted to other people when the façades are attractive. At least on first meeting, we are remembered by what we look like rather than by what we say or do.

Beauty is a state of mind, essentially—a confidence, a self-respect, a certain amount of common sense. There isn't a hairdresser in this world, including myself, who has the time or could charge the price it would take to really make a woman over—she must have the basic feeling of beauty, the essential good taste, because there's more to it than the mechanics. A beautiful woman is beautiful *before* her hairdo or her makeup, because she *feels* she is.

And beauty is habit—of the eye, the mind, the hand—that is very hard for people to change. Most women learn to do their makeup and hair styling early in their lives, perhaps even in high school. They find it extremely difficult to abandon their habits and can't visualize themselves looking any different.

Women constantly say to me, "I just can't get the hang of it," but I tell them to think of all the people they know who *can* cope with their hair or their makeup, who *can* make a change. They had to learn. So can you.

Chapter 3

HAIR CARE

Beautiful hair doesn't just happen. Beautiful hair is the result of total hair care. I think, in the next few years, we'll be seeing much more emphasis on the care and feeding of the hair and scalp, as we see more and more free, bouncy, natural heads of hair. Many people find this hard to understand because they are hung up on the idea that they need a hairdo that stays where it's put for a week. We simply have to reaccustom our eyes to new shapes and forms and new methods of doing things.

Many women start out with lovely hair. But if they do too little, if they just let it hang there without shaping, or conditioning or proper cleansing, it won't stay that way long. If they abuse it by doing too *much* to it, too much dyeing, too much straightening, too much sunning or permanenting or spraying, its beauty will disappear even faster.

People have, after all, only one head of hair. That's why it's so unbelievable to me that they do such incredibly weird things to it. They abuse it, torment it and wonder why it looks so terrible. Then they ask if there isn't a bottle of some magical stuff that will restore it once more. There isn't. If you destroy your hair by some excessive chemical process, nobody can help you do anything but hide it. If you break your hair off, it's gone. It just isn't there any more. If you don't understand hair coloring, for example, you may think you can lighten your hair and then go back to your natural color the next day if you don't like it. You can't. There is no natural way back. You have done something permanent to it, even if it took you only five minutes to do it.

If you are to have beautiful hair, your general health must be good. Your diet is important because the roots of the hair are nourished by the food you eat. Exercise is important. If your general condition isn't good, your hair will show it along with your skin and your nails. Even a cold can make your hair limp or oily or full of dandruff. Too little sleep has an effect, and so does excessive drinking and smoking. Anything detrimental to the body affects your hair. Even your mental state can change it.

Beneath every beautiful head of hair is a clean and healthy scalp. The most sensational hairdo ever created won't give you shimmering, touchable, real hair if the scalp below is grimy or in poor condition. It's like trying to grow beautiful flowers in poor, undernourished, neglected soil.

Right now I'm going to give you a short course in good hair care because I'm sure it's safe to say that you spend a lot of time on your hair style and remarkably little on its health.

Shampoos

Though I don't know a single woman who admits to giving herself a poor shampoo, I'd be willing to bet most of you don't really know how to do it right. There's more to it than water and a slathering of soap.

First of all, it doesn't matter how often you wash your hair. You should shampoo it whenever it's dirty. If that's every day, then it's every day. It won't hurt to wash it frequently and, in fact, it's much healthier to have clean hair than dirty hair.

If your hair doesn't get dirty quickly I'd suggest washing it once a week, even if it still looks all right. Oil and dirt do accumulate on the scalp and they don't have a very pleasant smell.

If your bangs and hairline get dirty before the rest of your hair and you don't feel like having a complete shampoo, you can wash them separately over the sink. Pin the rest of the hair back out of the way, wet the bangs and wash with shampoo. Now rinse thoroughly.

Shampoos are made for every variety of hair: normal, oily, dry, bleached, dandruffy, etc. Pick the one that seems to apply best to you and don't be afraid to switch around and experiment with different kinds. I've found that each head is unique, and different products will work in different ways on different heads. And sometimes a product will work beautifully for a while and then it won't. If you try something else for a few weeks and then go back, the results may be better.

I'd like to see people avoid shampoos that are really detergents because of their often caustic effect. Some shampoos, too, actually bleach the hair slightly each time you use them. How many times have you found, after using a certain shampoo for a couple of months, that your hair is a little lighter, maybe a little redder, and maybe a bit more brittle?

If your hair gets dirty too soon to be convenient, a dry shampoo may take out enough oil to make life bearable another day. It shouldn't, however, be used instead of a real shampoo on a regular basis. A dry shampoo can be helpful, too, for cleaning bangs or hairlines which show soil first.

Before you wet your hair to shampoo it, give it a good stiff brushing to activate the oil glands and loosen any dead scales on the scalp. Then massage the scalp gently with your fingertips, using a circular motion starting at the temples and working back to the nape. If your scalp is dry and you need a hot oil treatment, do it now.

Now thoroughly wet your hair with warm water. (If you've been using hair spray, give it a good rinse with very hot water.) Apply the shampoo. Vigorously massage your scalp, paying special attention to the hairline, with the rounded part of your fingertips, being careful not to use your fingernails. Use a soft plastic brush or a nailbrush in the hairline area, and be sure to scrub the scalp clean—without irritating it. If your hair is long, be sure that the ends are well soaped and washed—rub them together as you would your lingerie.

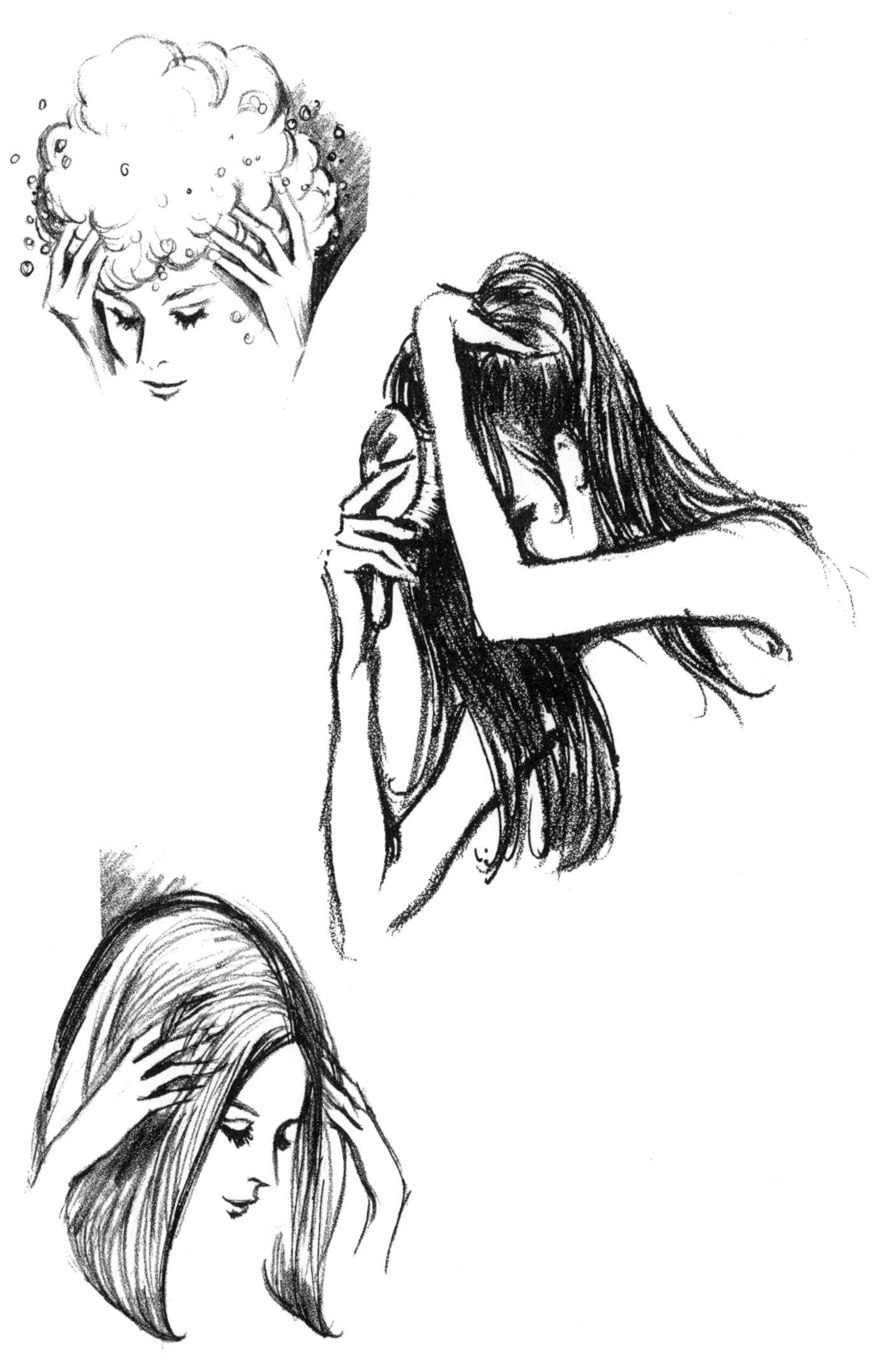

Now rinse madly. This is where most people go wrong. Soap left in the hair can be disaster. It leaves a dull film on it, makes it limp and droopy. If you do your shampooing in the shower, you'll find a good rinsing is easier.

After you're *sure* all the soap is out, rinse a few more times. One soaping is usually plenty, especially if your hair is normal or dry. Finally, if you can stand it, give your hair a rinse in cold water. I don't know why, but somehow this helps to give the hair a shine.

If you live in a hard-water area, you probably use a softener in your water system. If you don't, an easy solution for home use is to add a tablespoon of borax to a gallon of water and to give your hair a final rinse with this. There are also special soap-curd removers which you can add to the rinse water to take out any remains of the shampoo.

If you're going to use a special rinse—cream, color, etc.—do it now.

Wrap a towel around your head to soak up some of the water; towel-dry it as much as you can. Then comb it, starting at the ends and working up to the roots to get the tangles out.

(See Chapter 4 on "Problem Hair" if yours needs special care.)

Your brush and comb must be kept scrupulously clean, too.

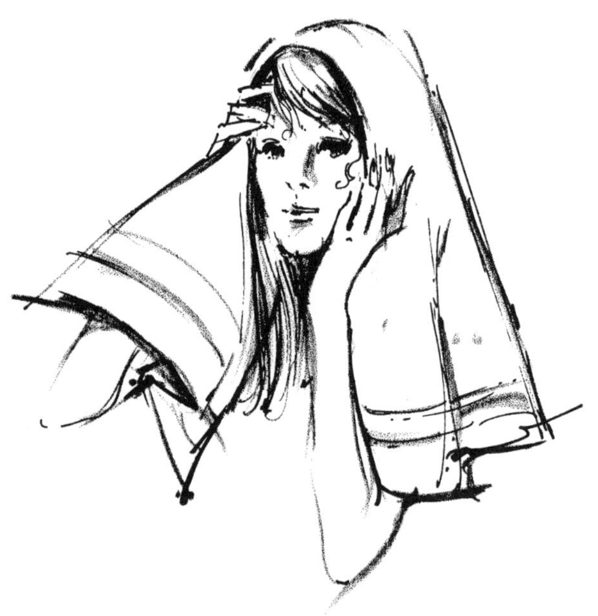

Clean them before you shampoo your hair. Wash in lukewarm soapy water (never a harsh detergent) with a little ammonia in it. Immerse only the bristles of the brush if the handle is not plastic. Your combs should be scrubbed with a nailbrush or left to soak for a while. Rinse well.

If your brush is made of natural bristle, dry it by wiping it gently on a rough turkish towel, then leave it in the open air with the bristles down on a clean towel. A plastic-bristle brush may merely be dried on a towel as the synthetic material does not absorb water.

By the way, it's only logical to keep *all* of your hair equipment clean. If you wash your hair regularly, why not wash the things that constantly touch your hair? Rollers. Hair clips. Hair nets. After all, they too get covered with setting lotion and hair spray and just plain dirt. They get sticky. Dunk them every so often in soapy water.

Scalp Care

Anything that urges blood to the head nourishes the scalp. Therefore, the second step to a healthy head is some kind of stimulation of the scalp itself to encourage circulation, which in turn helps to feed the hair follicles. You need this especially if your hair is dull and lifeless or dry or thin. (One warning: If you have an oily scalp, stimulation tends to increase oil production.)

Starting at the hairline, using all five fingers against the scalp,

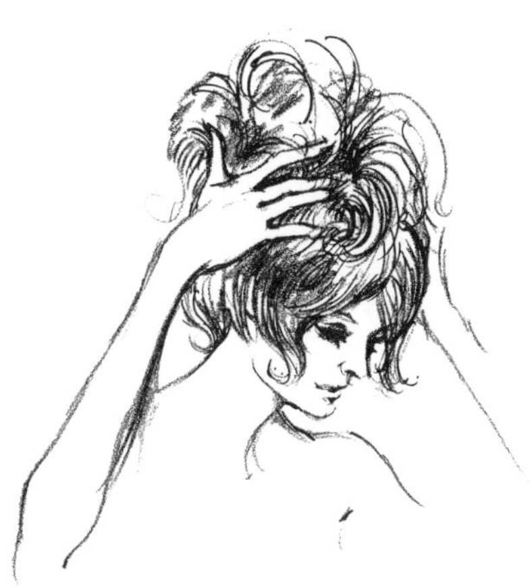

press lightly and massage in a circular motion, moving slowly back to the nape about a half inch at a time. If you have a cooperative husband or friend, enlist some help.

Always massage your scalp gently. Irritation of the skin is definitely not what you're after.

One of the best treatments for the scalp is a good brushing—every day—with a rounded bristle brush, again to encourage circulation and to help remove dust, dead scales and hair spray.

First, work out any tangles by gently brushing the ends of the hair; then brush another inch or so above the ends; then another inch, until the tangles are removed all the way to the scalp. Never, never yank or hack at your hair, because all you'll do is pull the hair out or break it. If you have an impossible tangle, it's often best to separate the hair carefully with your fingers before you start with the brush.

Now, lying on a bed with your head hanging over the edge, or sitting with your head bent way down, brush the hair from the nape up to the ends of the hair. Touch the scalp with the bristles, but never, never press hard enough to irritate the scalp. Use slow, smooth strokes.

Take some time out every day—about ten or fifteen minutes—to lie down with your head lower than the rest of your body. Or, if you can manage it, learn how to stand on your head. This will do wonders for your circulation, not only in your scalp but your face as well.

If you like using an electric vibrator on your scalp, that's fine, too. What you're after is better circulation because that means better hair.

Hot-Oil Treatments

If your scalp is exceedingly dry you could occasionally give it a hot-oil treatment. This used to be considered good for dry or damaged hair, but today, with the products that are available for conditioning your hair, it's pretty silly to try to do it with oil. Manufacturers have developed far more sophisticated and effective products for hair conditioning than a bottle of olive oil. They've spent millions developing conditioners for every conceivable variety of hair type, making oil absolutely archaic (unless, of course, you feel you *must* use only natural materials).

Hot-oil treatments are not archaic, however, for the scalp. They can help correct a dry scalp. Take about a quarter of a cup of oil—castor, olive, mineral, whatever—and heat it. Make it pretty hot but not so hot that you can't stand it. Make little parts all over your head, a section at a time, and, with a cotton pad, rub the oil into your scalp.

Now wrap steaming hot towels (dip them in very hot water and then wring them out—you may need rubber gloves) around your head. Or use a heat cap. Or sit under a hot dryer. Continue the heat for fifteen or twenty minutes. If you prefer, leave the oil on overnight with your hair wrapped up so the oil doesn't get all over your pillow. I would like to think you'd do this only if you sleep alone and you don't care what you look like all night long.

Now rinse your hair in very hot water for a few minutes. Give it enough sudsings—at the very least, two—to get all the oil out. Castor oil, though considered one of the best, is the hardest to remove.

Cream Rinses

The cream rinse was one of the first hair conditioners and it certainly has its place and benefits. But remember that when you use a cream rinse, you are softening the hair, reducing its natural body, while at the same time making it easy, in its wet stage, to comb out tangles. Cream rinses are a great help if your hair is coarse and stiff, or dry and strawlike, and what you need is the softening effect. It's good for hair that is frizzy and tangles easily—if it is coarse. But for other hair, especially fine, limp hair, cream rinses will make the whole situation much worse by removing whatever body your hair does have.

If your hair is fine, even if it's frizzy, I'd prefer to struggle a little more and skip the cream rinse. If you feel you *must* use it because your hair tangles that badly, then do it this way: When you put on the rinse, comb your hair straight and smooth with a wide-toothed comb. Comb it straight back if you're doing the job in the shower; comb it forward if you're doing it over the sink. Then *thoroughly* rinse out the cream rinse, using plenty of hot water, applying the water in the same direction that you've combed. This will cut down on some of the softening action of the cream and still get some of the tangles out.

By the way, hairdressers or shampoo girls often automatically put a cream rinse on the hair after a wash. If you don't want it, warn them in advance not to use it on you.

Instead of a cream rinse, the old-fashioned vinegar rinse works very well on some tangly hair. Take a jigger of vinegar, mix it in a cup of water and pour it through the hair after a shampoo. Rinse well.

Hair Conditioners

You can temporarily improve the appearance of your hair and give it some protection by the use of conditioners. Conditioners will not cure damaged or poor hair, but they can help it to look and behave better from shampoo to shampoo. Conditioners are designed simply to coat the hair, smoothing out the hair shaft and/or acting as a filler for the hair shaft. When hair is damaged, the cuticle or outer layer has often been broken or pitted, making each hair tangle on the next one. Or the hair has become extremely porous or dried out, or broken or split. The proper conditioner can disguise the damage, making it look better and easier to handle. It *temporarily,* from shampoo to shampoo, will replace some of the oils and proteins that have been removed.

There are as many kinds of conditioners as there are hair prob-

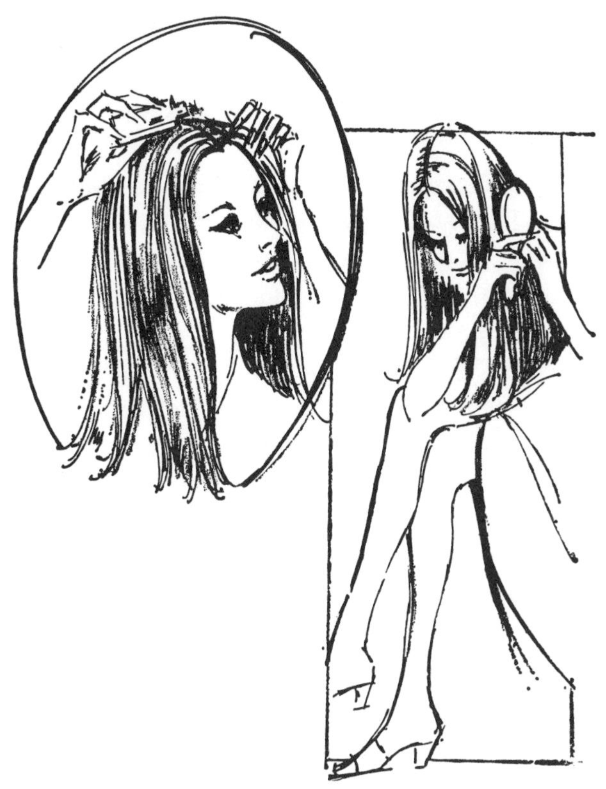

lems. As with a shampoo, choose the one which seems best suited to your hair, and don't hesitate to switch around from kind to kind and brand to brand. You may choose one that is merely a conditioner, or it may be combined with a shampoo or even with setting lotion or hair spray. The more severe hair problems require a pure conditioner. Each product has its own specific directions—follow them exactly.

Conditioners come in two basic types:

CORRECTIVE CONDITIONERS: These smooth out the damaged hair shaft and disguise the problem, replacing for the moment some of the oils and proteins. These are usually worked into the hair after a shampoo, left on for a time (from a few seconds to a half hour), and then rinsed out. A few products are designed to be left in without rinsing or even used as a setting lotion.

Use a conditioner as often as you feel it's necessary, every shampoo if you like.

Because conditioners add oil, they are hardly what you need if your hair is oily. They will make it oilier. If, however, your *scalp* is oily but your *hair* is dry, damaged or brittle from being treated shabbily, then you should use a conditioner but apply it *only* to the *hair,* not to the scalp.

If your hair is fine and limp, avoid a conditioner with a cream base which will soften it more. Read the label or look at the consistency. Does it look creamy and slippery or does it look watery? If it's like water, it's obviously not cream.

To eliminate surface dirt from dry hair, you occasionally can use a conditioner instead of a shampoo—wet the hair, apply the conditioner and rinse out.

BODYBUILDERS OR TEXTURIZERS: The bodybuilders are essentially "fillers." These penetrate the hair shaft and give each hair more substance, as well as making it smoother and less porous. Many contain protein which is designed to coat the damaged hair shaft and make it sleeker and shinier. The idea is to build up volume and body in thin, limp, droopy hair.

These work quite well, especially the first couple of times you use them. But they do have a tendency—after prolonged use—to dry out the hair or to build up on the hair, making it start to snap off. I suggest using the bodybuilders, if they help you, for two weeks at a time, then laying off for a few weeks.

Most texturizers are applied after the shampoo and not rinsed out.

Summer Care

It has always seemed madness to me that women spend their summers neglecting their hair or tormenting it with sun, wind, salt water and chlorine. Then after Labor Day they rush out to buy lotions, potions and magic elixirs they hope will bring it back to its glorious natural condition in one easy swoop.

It just doesn't work. You can help your hair once you've abused it, but it won't really recover until you've grown a whole new crop.

Why not avoid all the problems and take care of it during the summer instead?

Cover your hair in the sun, especially if it's been tinted, bleached, permanented or straightened. The sun can lighten natural hair, and completely change the color of color-treated hair, turning it brassy or dull or red. The sun will also dry your hair out, causing split ends and breakage as well as turning it into a reasonable facsimile of straw, particularly if it's been chemically treated. Wear a scarf over it or a brimmed hat whenever you're outside.

Don't leave salt water, chlorinated pool water or suntan lotions in your hair. When you come in from the beach or the pool and rinse yourself off, rinse your hair out too. A shampoo is even better, along with an instant conditioner which you leave on for a minute before washing out.

Conditioners are particularly important in the summertime—I suggest using them with every shampoo if your hair is dry. And why not, if you lead a concentrated beach life, put a conditioner on your hair *before* you go to the beach? Your hair will get wet anyway, and under the head covering, it won't be seen.

Cut your hair regularly in summer, at least once every four weeks—it grows faster in warm weather.

Try to avoid excessive hair spray. In humid air it tends to get sticky.

Moisturize your skin at every opportunity. You can't do it too often. And I believe everyone, whether she burns or not, should use a sun-filtering agent. Get a deep tan every year and at forty or forty-five you'll have a crinkled, dried-out, shoe-leather face looking back at you from the mirror. Americans tend to admire tans and certainly most of us look better with some color—but sun is the skin's and hair's worst enemy.

Obviously, the simplest, easiest hair style is best for summer. Just about every client I see wants one that requires minimum care and won't look awful when it isn't set. To me, that means short wash-and-wear hair, or long wash-and-wear hair, perhaps with the help of a hairpiece.

The ideal short drip-dry hair doesn't need setting at all, but can be combed into place. Comb some setting lotion through your hair after you've towel-dried it, just for body to hold it in line while it dries completely. Or blow it dry, using a brush and a hand dryer to create a bit of volume. Or put a few rollers on the top if you want some bounce.

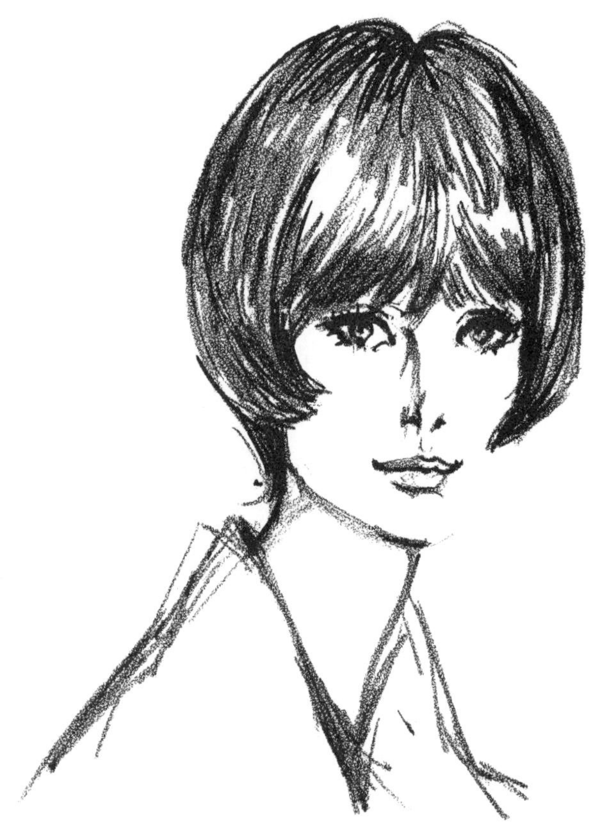

Wash-and-wear styles have to be very simple and you can't expect always to get the most flattering look for yourself. But that's not too important when you think about the convenience of hair that looks neat and is easy to cope with at the beach. You don't want to have to run for the hairdresser or your curlers every time you climb out of the water.

If you don't look good in a short style, why not a long one, just as easy to cope with. When I talk about long hair, I don't mean way down to there. Hair longer than three or four inches below the shoulders is difficult to handle until you have the knack for it. The hair length I think looks best ranges from an inch below the chin to four inches below the shoulders. It should be essentially all one length, or a little longer in front, so you can contain it in some way in the back.

You can wear this length free, in braids or pulled back in a pony-tail. Longer hair makes it easier to add simple hairpieces, such as an extra braid or a wiglet done in curls. If you want a dressier look for evening, the classic French twist is quite elegant.

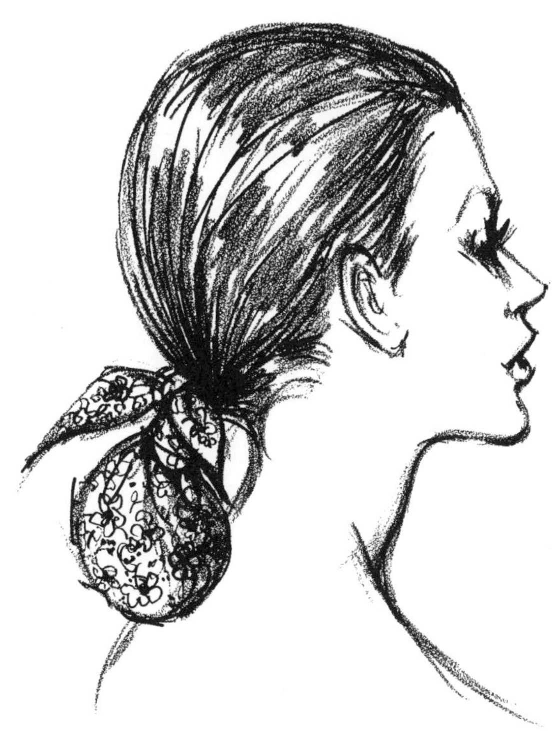

And don't forget wigs for summer. They can be your answer.

If you have a problem with frizzy hair in the summer, you can find a few possible solutions in "Frizzy Hair," Chapter 4.

For fine hair that droops, see "Fine Hair" in Chapter 4. Perhaps a body wave is what you need.

Winter Care

If you're an avid skier, you've probably got a hair problem unless you wear your hair in a wash-and-wear style—short and shaped so it will look presentable when there is no set at all. Or long, so you can hold it back in some way. Skiing is very rough on the hair. Usually you wear a cap or a hood which is guaranteed to destroy any coiffure in half an hour. Your hair either gets stuck to your head or

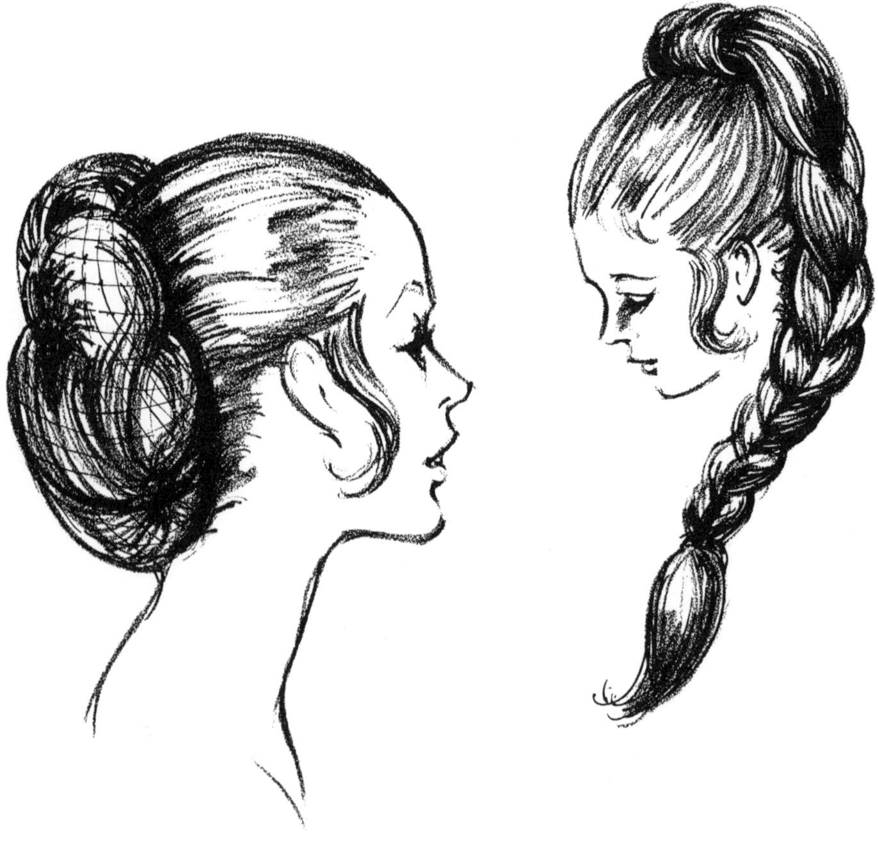

it turns dry and electric and stands out on end when you take off your hat. If you can't just comb it into some kind of line, I suggest you carry a kerchief in your pocket to put on when you go in for lunch. Then wash your hair before dinner.

At night, when you want to look pretty, give yourself a quick hairdo with heated rollers, or a curling iron, or a wig, a wiglet or other hairpiece, if the wash-and-wear thing doesn't work for you.

Even non-sportswomen have winter troubles. If you keep your head under cover all the time, your hair may become too oily too soon—you'll have to wash it whenever it needs it. If it suffers from static electricity, a cream rinse might be helpful along with a light film of hair spray.

The Tools You'll Need

There is always something else to buy, something else that supposedly will turn you magically into a great beauty who has no trouble at all with her hair. Frankly, I think too many "beauty aids" are really just gimmicks and I don't see any need for them. If they make you feel better, fine, but you can get along beautifully with just the basics.

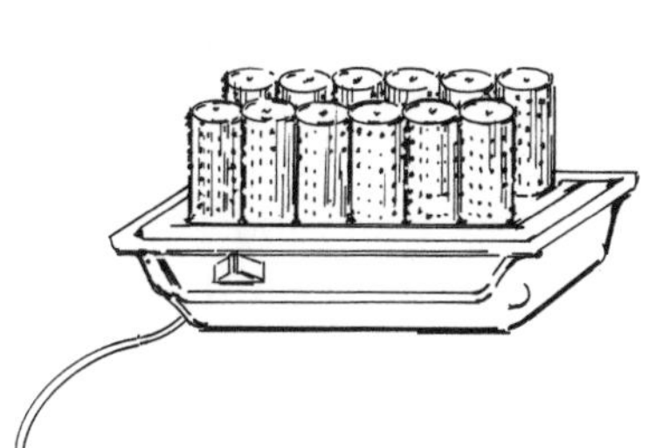

BRUSHES: I don't think it matters whether you have a natural-bristle brush or a synthetic one. In salons, we can't even consider natural bristle because, with the constant washing after each client, it doesn't hold up. The anti-nylon brush syndrome, which says you must never use a synthetic but always a natural bristle, is no longer valid anyway. Natural bristle is very nice, but the objections to synthetics have been overcome. In the early days, when nylon brushes were made as cheap replacements for the real thing, the bristles were cut off straight and sharp and had a terrible tendency to irritate the scalp as well as to catch and break the hair. Today, however, they can be very much like the natural—tapered and smooth and fine for the hair.

The way to choose a brush is, first, to be sure the bristles are rounded. Then choose according to the shape which feels most comfortable to you—it really doesn't matter. I happen to like those with a rubbery air cushion base because the "give" makes them conform better to the shape of the head. If your hair is very thick and coarse, look for a brush that is big and strong and deep. Thin, fine hair hardly needs an enormous brush. Find the comfortable one for you.

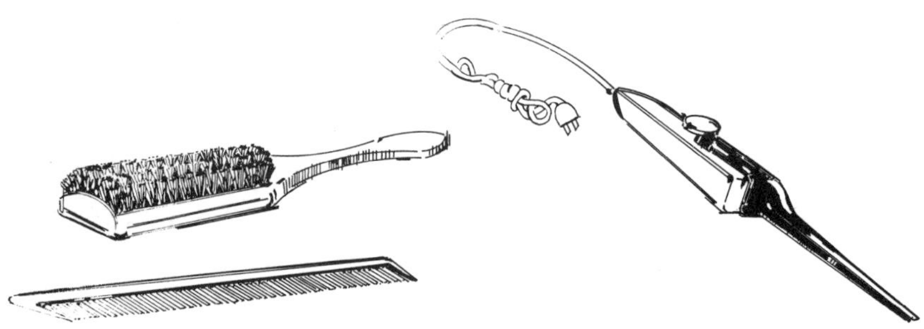

COMBS: Again, anything that's comfortable for you is perfectly all right, as long as it has smooth tips and doesn't scratch the head. I prefer a comb with both wide and narrow teeth, and I happen to like the hard rubber kind because they are easier on the hair and last longer since they don't snap in two as easily as plastic. They have more bend to them. Use the wide-toothed part to comb out wet tangles. I don't think I've had a rattail comb in my hand for ten years, but many people find them handy for sectioning the hair for setting, and for lifting it after combing to give some height. For lift, I happen to like a long stiff hairpin.

CLIPS: Just remember to discard them when the springiness is gone.

BOBBY PINS: No problem here. All bobby pins, I assume, are rubber- or plastic-tipped now, and slide into the hair easily. If the tips break off or if the coating on the bobby pins wears away, throw them out.

END PAPERS: Always use these to cover the ends of the hair when you roll them up. They make the ends smoother, prevent hooking and eliminate stray wisps.

ROLLERS: Rollers come in many sizes. If your hair is long or very curly, or you want a very loose set, use the biggest ones. Most women need a variety—the larger ones for the crown and back, smaller ones for the hairline area. My favorite kind of roller is the wire mesh because I feel it is easiest on the hair and easiest to work with. I definitely object to the brush rollers because they scratch the scalp and snag the hair; magnetic rollers slip and slide too much; the soft foam "sleep" rollers don't work because they do not provide enough tension; plastic rollers are more difficult than the wire mesh to clip securely.

Keep your rollers clean by washing them now and then. After constant use, they become sticky and dirty just like your hair.

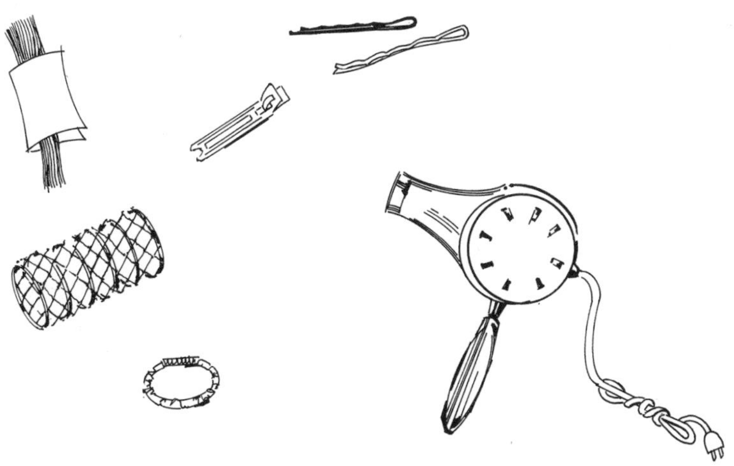

CURLING IRONS: These should never be used to style a head of hair from scratch, but only to touch up a set. If a curl loosens or straightens, and when there is not time to do a whole set or to heat up some heated rollers, the curling iron will do the job. Use it quickly without leaving the heat on the hair for more time than it takes to produce the curl.

Another handy use for a curling iron is to straighten out curly hair. You take the iron and pull the hair through it, stretching out the curl, literally ironing it straighter.

ELECTRIC ROLLERS: There are so many varieties of electric rollers on the market today that it is hard to make a choice. I would choose according to the hair style you wear. Some sets come with rollers all one size: small, medium or large. Some sets have mixed sizes. Some have only six or eight rollers; others have up to twenty. My preference would be a larger set, so you'll be sure to have enough for your hair, and one with mixed sizes as you'll sometimes want a tighter curl somewhere, perhaps at the nape. The very small roller sets are, of course, lighter weight for traveling, and they're good for girls who never want more than a few curls.

ELASTICS: Never use a plain rubber band on your hair. It will snarl it, break it, split it. Use covered elastics. Sometimes I take a piece of narrow ribbon and tie it around in place of the elastic. This works well if the hair isn't exceptionally fine and wispy.

HAIR DRYERS: The salon-type dryers with the rigid hoods are very useful if you set your hair at home in the conventional way. They will dry the hair much more quickly than the air will, and make for a set that lasts longer.

I think a hand dryer is a necessity too, to semi-dry the hair before a set, or to give yourself a blow-dry hairdo. Make sure it has plenty of air and heat power, and is quite comfortable to hold in your hand for the time it takes for your hair to dry.

The bonnet-type dryers, while maybe better than nothing, do not usually allow enough air circulation to dry the hair evenly, especially if you use very large rollers.

Chapter 4

PROBLEM HAIR

Just about every woman who ever walks into my salon thinks she has a hair problem. What's more, hers is unique. Her hair is finer than anyone else's could possibly be. Or nobody's hair is quite as kinky as hers. In the last twenty years, I think I've talked about fine hair and kinky hair and oily hair so much—in print as well as in person—that it seems to me everyone in the United States must have heard all the answers. But I still get letter after letter and question after question from women who have problems with their hair.

Each person looks for instant magic. There *must* be something in a bottle, tube or jar that will make her hair beautiful, manageable and suitable for whatever the current hair style may be. Well, there are all kinds of temporary aids today, but you have to keep in mind that none of them are permanent and that, usually, you are stuck with your problem.

It seems to me that what you must do is really understand your particular hair problem, and then try to find a good basic approach to it. You have to start with that. Take, for example, fine hair. Women with baby-fine hair too often want to take this baby-fine hair and turn it into something that is architecturally impossible for it to keep longer than half an hour, unless it's sprayed into a concrete block. Then they go on complaining about how their fine hair won't hold a set. Of course it won't. Accept that and have it cut in a good shape that will look presentable without any set at all. That's the best advice I can give, the most logical approach. It may not make you happy, like the advice that very oily hair must be washed whenever it's dirty, maybe every day, but it's the only honest thing I can say to you.

Right now I think everybody's lucky because the best-looking hair is not being worn in elaborate puffed-up shapes. It's much more natural. A woman with fine hair can wear it straight and swinging and look great. A girl whose excessively curly hair has always obsessed her can forget about straightening it and let it go absolutely kinky and wonderful with the right haircut. This may require a whole change of eye and a lot of people can't make that change, but if you can you're much better off. The way you wear your hair —and apply your makeup—really becomes a habit. But habits can be changed and should be if you come to realize that the hairdo you've been wearing, or the techniques you've been using on it, aren't suitable to your own particular head of hair.

Now here are some specific problems and the basic solutions I've found to be the best for them.

Fine Hair

I hear complaints about fine hair every day of the week and I sympathize. Every woman would like to set her hair once a week and have it look terrific till the next time. But if she has fine hair it just isn't going to work out that way.

Fine hair is fine in texture and therefore much harder to manage than coarser hair. It has a tendency to fly around and not hold a curl. It splits and breaks more easily, it separates, it can be adversely affected by excessive coloring, harsh shampoos, straightening and any other chemical process that can be detrimental to hair. It feels everything first. It flattens down easily. It is full of static electricity.

Fine hair cannot be forced into unnatural shapes without the use of strong permanents, excessive hair spray and a lot of teasing. And the owner ends up with hair that is brittle, dry, broken, thin, sticky and generally unattractive. Luckily, for all of you with this kind of hair, we seem to be emerging from the era of concrete hairdos. If you wear your hair loose and swinging, you'll do great.

First, you need—absolutely—a blunt cut done with scissors. This is crucial. I'm not even going to insist that the hair must be all one length, though I think it's easier to cope with on a daily basis.

If your hair is *thin* as well as fine, it *must* be a blunt, all-one-length hair style. I know all the other answers: layering, permanenting, setting on smaller rollers, etc., but I have to tell you that twenty-five years of working on this problem has proved to me that you can't have the best of all possible worlds, ever. You can't always please yourself, your husband, your friends and your hair texture at the same time.

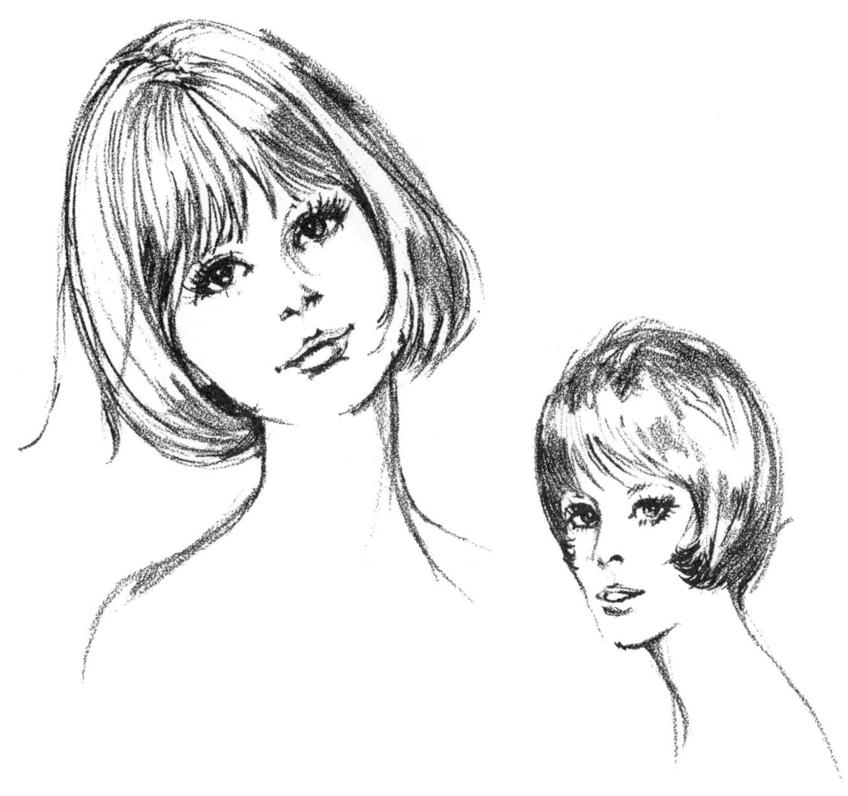

So again, thin fine hair needs the blunt even cut. Then you can set it if you like, but when it collapses—which it will—it will still have a good shape. If you just can't accept this answer, then why don't you grow your hair long and wear it in a French twist or a chignon? Or wrap up the long hair, and use a hairpiece or even a wig for part of the week when you don't want to fuss.

If your hair is fine but quite heavy and thick, *then* it can be layered if you like.

If you want some curl or turn to your hair, or some very definite line, have some sort of soft permanent wave, either a body wave or more, depending on the hair style you wear, the weight and the length of your hair. In general, you'll find that your hair will keep a better shape if it is shorter than long because the weight of long hair makes it droop.

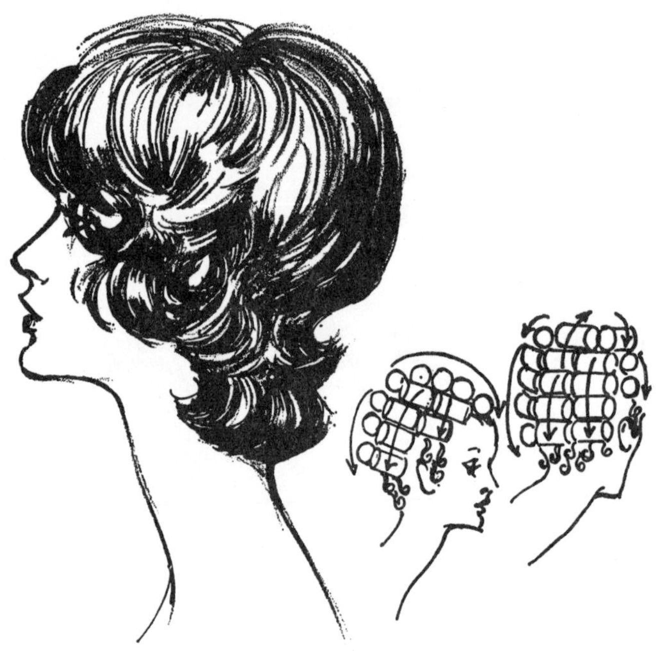

Then, find a good "extra hold" setting lotion that gives a great deal of body. Fortunately we no longer use the old quince- and flax-based gooey setting lotions that used to leave such a residue on the hair. Even beer, which so many people used for so long, is no longer necessary with the development of new kinds of lotions in the last few years.

Always remember that a product that works on one person's hair may not work on another's. So keep experimenting until you find one that works well for you.

One helpful hint: This is something I do very often when I have a client with extremely fine hair. Dry the hair with a hand dryer after the shampoo and then apply the setting lotion. This way the water won't dilute the lotion and it will hold even better.

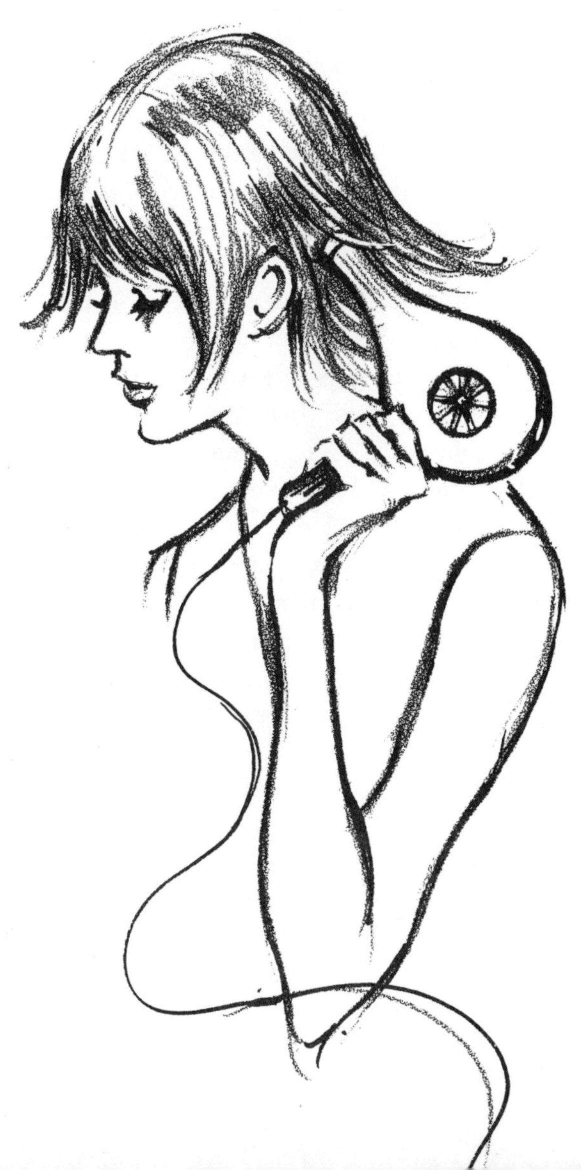

Keep your fine hair in good condition by using a *non*-cream conditioner regularly, though if your hair is oily remember that conditioners might encourage too much oiliness.

Some people have good results with texturizers or bodybuilders, but I've found that consistent use can make the hair seem too dry and even cause some breaking. I suggest using them once or twice, then laying off for a couple of weeks before starting again.

Never, never use any product which has a cream base on your fine hair. Never use a cream rinse. It will make your hair even softer and limper.

Sometimes coloring can add a certain amount of body to fine hair. Streaking can help if you don't want all-over color and for most people it is probably the better solution. Remember to avoid the temporary coloring products that have cream bases.

Fine hair will have more body and keep its set longer if you use smaller rollers, wrapping the ends with paper. Then back-comb the hair just a little when you brush it out. But if your hair is terribly fine or terribly thin, it will come out too tight and kinky this way and will look even thinner. In this case, you will be better off if you leave the hair loose with just a slight turn in it.

Use a light hair spray, and never overdo it. I stay away from the hair sprays that say "extra hold" because they seem to make the hair appear stiff and unreal. Besides, what's so wrong if your hair does blow around a little bit? If you've got a good haircut, a quick combing will put it back in place.

Just remember, whatever you do, your set won't last a week as it might for someone with coarse hair.

I hate to say this but your hair will probably keep its shape best with a professional set, so have it done when you can spend the money. It holds better for many reasons: more roller tension, smoother curling, heat drying, better comb-out. If you pay attention to how your hair is done by a professional, maybe your home settings will improve.

I'd suggest the acquisition of a fall in a simple, slightly turned-under version to wear between settings. And perhaps a wig for the times when all else fails.

The really final solution, besides hairpieces, is probably to grow your hair long and wrap it up, perhaps in a French twist or a chignon, so you don't have to worry at all about getting volume. This kind of solution sometimes gives you a very definitive style which can become your own trade-mark, an individuality that is great to have even though it comes about as an answer to the problem of terribly fine hair.

Oily Hair

This is the other most common complaint hairdressers hear from their clients. And I'm sorry to say, it often goes together with fine hair.

Everyone's scalp secretes oil, of course, but some people have so much oil that their hair is soiled only a day or so after a shampoo, not only because of the oil but because the oil collects soot and dust. I can sympathize with these people because I have the same problem myself—oily, thin hair that must be washed every day if I'm to look like I have any hair at all.

Whether you like it or not, you too must wash your hair every day, if necessary, or as often as it soils. That is the Number One treatment and is essential. There are shampoos especially made for you which help to cut the oil. Wash with warm water, not hot.

Then there is the thing of using lemon. This is rather an old wives' remedy but it can help. Squeeze a fresh lemon, dilute the juice in a cup of lukewarm water and pour it over your hair after shampooing. Leave it for five minutes and then rinse out with cooler water. Remember, however, that the natural action of lemon can lighten the hair a shade or two. Vinegar makes another rinse for oily hair. Mix it with water and use after the shampoo. Rinse out.

A helpful trick that may sound crazy but it works for lots of people is an icy cold rinse after a shampoo.

If your hair is so oily that it is stringy by the middle of the day after washing it, it seems to me you ought to wash it in the morning instead of the night before, so you get through a complete day looking good.

Never dry your hair under a hot dryer but turn it on warm and finish off with cool air.

Between shampoos, you can use a dry shampoo, following the directions for the specific product. Usually it is applied, then the hair is gently brushed with a *clean* brush which is wiped on a towel between strokes.

Another way to remove some oil between washings is to pour a little cologne on a piece of cotton and wipe the scalp with it. Work only on the hairline or your bangs if that's all you need, or section off the hair and rub the saturated cotton pad along the scalp.

Some people find it helps to cover their brush with a piece of clean gauze and brush with that to remove some of the excess oil.

These in-between cleanings can be useful, but, if your hair is so oily that it looks it, WASH IT.

Wash your comb and brush every time you wash your hair. If you don't, you'll be brushing oil right back into your clean hair. And don't brush too much. This will only carry the oil from your scalp down to the ends of the hair. Start the brushing a couple of inches from the scalp.

Probably your skin is oily too, and you must keep it scrupulously clean. Wash your face at least twice a day and more if possible. I don't think that's asking too much. First use a makeup remover, then wash your face and use astringent or toner for the pores.

If you have oily hair, especially if it's fine too, you should consider as simple a hair style as possible, one that really requires no setting and where the style is all in the cut and the shape, probably a shortish blunt cut. I prefer short hair because then the washing and drying aren't such a chore, though some women prefer long hair which they can pull up in some contained fashion. The blow-dry haircuts are perfect for oily-haired people.

If your problem is extremely severe, a visit to the doctor won't hurt. Sometimes ultraviolet treatments or injections of estrogen, for example, are recommended.

Cheer up—oily hair is a nuisance but it's the best kind to have in the long run. Oily hair doesn't break and split and dry out as

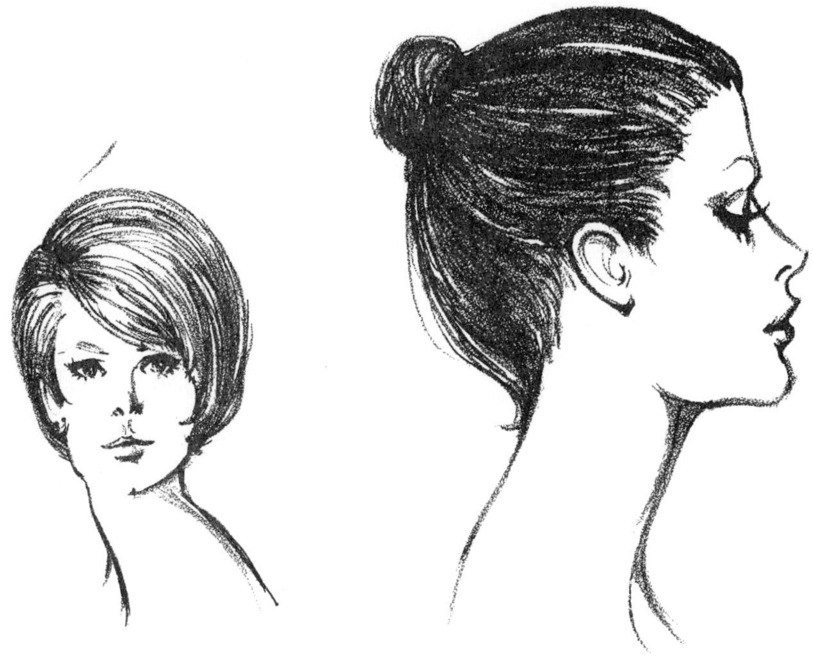

much as dry hair. And it means you probably have oily skin which will have better tone and won't wrinkle early—you'll be the envy of your dry-skinned friends. Besides, oily hair is usually a problem of the young. As you get older, the excessive oiliness will usually tend to disappear.

By the way, if your scalp is oily, a conditioner is probably *not* what you need because it will make your hair even oilier and slicker. But if your hair has become dry and strawlike (through abuse) even though your scalp is still oily, then a conditioner can be helpful. Avoid the kind with a cream base; look for one with a watery texture. Be sure you apply it to the hair only, *not* to your scalp.

To try to minimize the oiliness of your hair, stay away from butter, chocolate, nuts, fried foods, etc.

I've discovered that when I'm feeling tired and rather seedy, or when I have a cold, my hair gets oily much more quickly. Enough rest and attention to the general condition of the body is part of the treatment.

Thin Hair

One terrible and almost insoluble problem for many people is very, very thin hair. I'm talking about hair that is so sparsely spaced that the scalp actually shows through. This may be the result of heredity or illness or extreme emotional stress, a high fever, a malfunctioning thyroid gland. It can occur after a pregnancy. It can result from a poor diet or poor health. Sometimes no one knows the reason for it. And the hair gradually thins as one gets older.

Some thinness is caused by too much strain and stress on the hair, such as excessive brushing, too much teasing or pulling into a tight ponytail. Brush rollers are one of the great irritations, to my mind. Perhaps it's a temporary situation caused by overbleaching or overpermanenting. In this case, you're lucky because your hair will grow out again eventually and you'll have another chance to treat it better. Other people must learn to live with thin hair forever.

I'm afraid there are very few answers to this problem that will please you. There's not an awful lot you can do about it, but here are the answers that have worked best in my experience.

First, I believe in a basic kind of haircut, blunt cut and short, no longer than somewhere between the ear lobe and the chin, depending on your age. Then perhaps some kind of bangs coming from rather far back on the top of the head so that other people will not be looking right into the hairline—a dead giveaway for sparse hair.

This hair must be cut very carefully and very well so that it can be washed often. Thin hair must be scrupulously clean always so that it will have some volume, and perhaps be blown dry rather than set. You must avoid tight settings at all costs. Many people with thin hair tend to overcurl it because they think that makes it look thicker. I don't agree. I think excessive curliness can accent the look of thinness and a better solution for you is the simple blow-dry haircut.

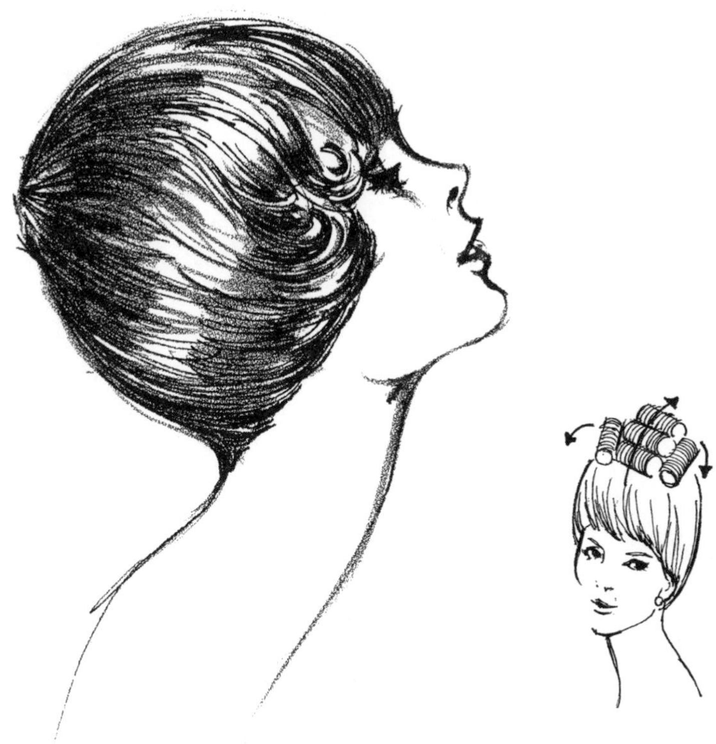

Another interesting approach to this problem, if you have the right coloring and are the right age, is to color your hair a warm shade of blond to make it look thicker. The reason this works is that the scalp is white or slightly pink and shows least through warm blond hair. However, a caution—if you are actually *losing* hair, I don't think you should color it.

If your hair is thin, put as little stress on it as possible. If you go to a hairdresser, ask him not to put too much tension on the rollers. Never use brush rollers. Never sleep on your rollers. Don't overbrush your hair. In fact, some dermatologists insist on absolutely no brushing if you have a problem. Don't overtease your hair. Don't pull it back tightly in a ponytail or chignon. Go easy with the hair spray and anything else you put on it. If your hair is falling, do nothing chemical to it—no coloring, no permanents, nothing. Your hair has enough troubles—don't add to them.

When you're out in the summer sun, keep your head covered. Russian doctors have reported that hair loss occurs mainly in the fall after a summer of sun beating down on an unprotected scalp.

Learn to stand on your head, or at least to lie on a slant board with your head lower than your body. This is a good way to help the circulation in the scalp, which could be your problem. So is an old-fashioned scalp massage, done with ten gentle fingers.

I realize that for some women wearing a wig or a hairpiece seems to be the ultimate defeat. But hairpieces are so attractive and versatile today that you should give them some serious thought. Not very long ago, wigs were in the same category as dentures or

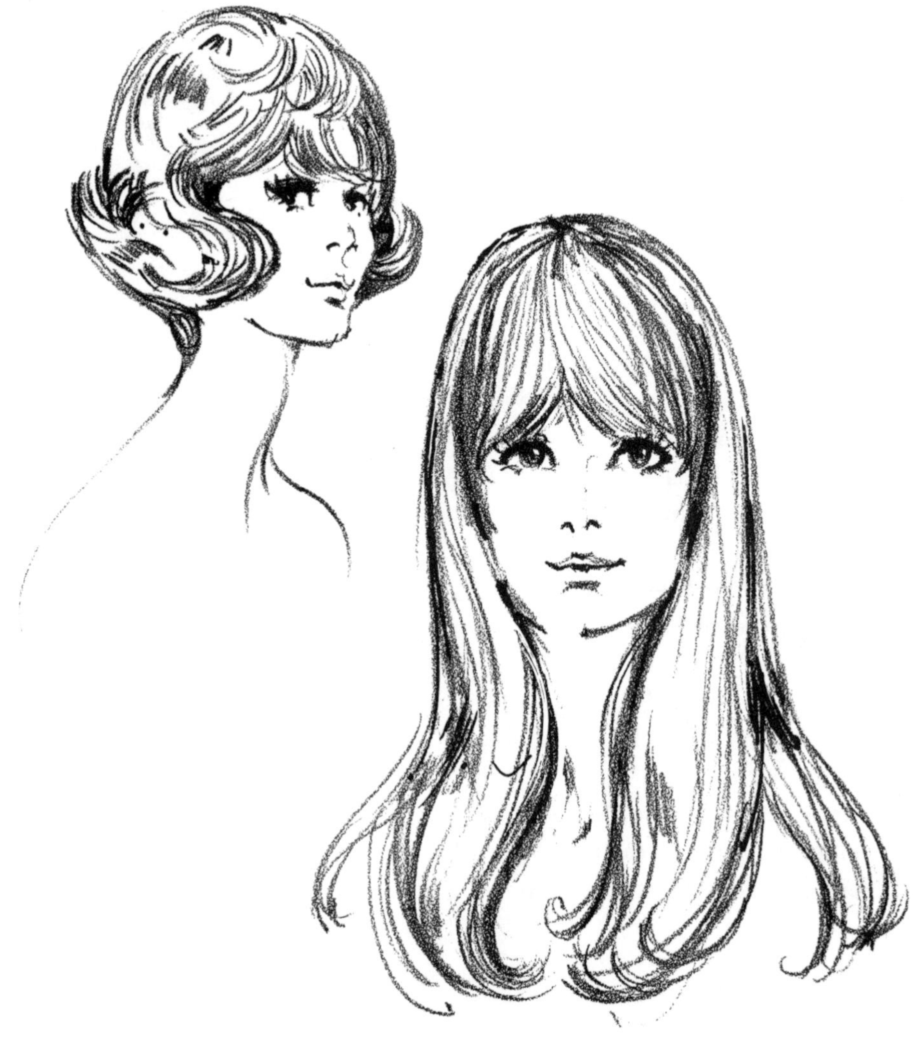

wooden legs, but now they're really genuine beauty aids. Women without your problem use them; certainly there's no stigma any more.

If you buy a wig, be sure it's very close to your own natural hair color and doesn't have a lot of bulk. You'll feel strange and you'll look strange with a sudden huge head of hair. Wearing a wig shouldn't worsen the condition of your own hair—certainly nobody wears a wig twenty-four hours a day.

Perhaps a small hairpiece would be all you need, maybe one that attaches just behind your hairline or on the top of your head to serve as a filler. Just don't wear it always in the same position; change the anchoring spot each time you put it on.

Falling Hair

I've talked about thin hair, but now I want to talk about hair that is actively and noticeably falling out. In these times when hair is so very important, to both men and women, anyone whose hair is departing from her head is probably more miserable about it than ever. These are times for thick, luxurious hair.

Don't be alarmed about a few hairs in your brush—everyone loses up to about one hundred hairs a day. The oldest hairs on your head are three to five years of age. When they reach maturity, which differs for everyone, they drop out and are replaced by new ones, growing at a rate of about a half inch per month.

But if you are losing more hair than you are replacing, and your hair is become noticeably thinner, then you should promptly try to find out if there is any physical reason for it. Go to your doctor. It could quite possibly be a result of some other condition of your body. I've found that actively falling hair can be caused by pregnancy, stopping the pill, a thyroid condition, the use of antibiotics, a very high fever or long illness, an estrogen deficiency, or an emotional crisis. Any change in the body can affect the hair, even a common cold.

Often, during pregnancy, women experience an accelerated surge of hair growth. Then, a couple of months after the delivery, they may lose a lot of hair within a short time and perhaps end up with thin hair. Almost always, these hairs are quickly replaced and there is no problem. Once in a while, it remains thin and only a doctor can tell her what she can possibly do about it.

I'm not the expert on these physical problems. Your doctor is. Don't fool around.

By the way, if you feel you'd like to see a dermatologist and you don't know one, call the local chapter of the AMA (American Medical Association) for recommendations, or ask your doctor.

I can't give medical advice. But I can speak from my experience as a hairdresser, and I'll tell you a few helpful hints. If your hair is actively falling out (and you've gone to the right doctor about it), treat it as gingerly as you can. Have it cut into a short simple blow-dry style that requires no rollers, no pin curls, no spraying, no anything. Stay away from *all* chemical processes such as coloring and permanenting. Do whatever your doctor suggests medically.

Put no stress on your hair. Comb and brush it gently. Don't tease it. Never pull it back tightly in a ponytail or bun. Never let the sun beat down on your unprotected head.

If your doctor approves—and be *sure*— it might be a good idea for you to buy a wig, one that's close to your own hair color and isn't too big and bulky. A smaller hairpiece would not be a good idea for you to use, because it must be firmly attached to your own hair and that would place too much stress on it.

Very Curly Hair

I happen to think curly hair can be beautiful. If it's cut properly, it is pretty and natural and individual. In the last ten years or so, fashion has leaned toward a straight look to the hair and consequently women with curly hair have found it the bane of their existence. Recently, however, the honesty of one's own curly hair has become more attractive along with the more individualized look of fashion in general. Witness, for example, the wearing of the Afro or the natural by many black people and how beautiful that can be.

But a lot of women just don't like their curly hair, and if they don't like it, they don't have to have it. They can have it straightened. (See Chapter 8.)

Some hair can be made completely straight; other hair can be relaxed somewhat but never made fully straight. Very fine curly hair, for example, will never become perfectly straight. To get it that way could seriously damage it. Incidentally, coarse hair is the easiest and safest to straighten, and the toughest section of hair of any texture to work on is around the crown and the hairline.

Sometimes the whole head needn't be straightened. It's possible to do it just at the hairline if this area tends to be particularly curly. We do this very often; in fact, we prefer to do only this section if that's all that's really needed because straightening often removes the natural body of the hair which the natural curl provides.

I never like to suggest that one should always go to a hairdresser. But in the case of straightening, I think it's much the best idea. There are good products made for home use, but I find that people have a terrible tendency not to read directions carefully. Remember that the chemical makeup of many hair straighteners is similar to the chemical makeup of a depilatory. That should tell you how very careful you must be—especially if you have fine hair.

Straightening should be done *at most* twice a year, and then always *before* a touch-up if you color your hair. Never, never do both the same day but wait at least a week for the touch-up. I've found that the chemicals in straighteners often remove some of the color even from natural hair. Do *not* attempt to straighten hair that's been colored with a two-process tint because it will be much too hard on it. Always be sure that the straightening does not overlap an old job as this double dose of the chemicals can be disastrous.

Have your hair straightened only when you really need it, when your hair is really unmanageable or it makes you miserable. Use a conditioner after every shampoo and go easy with the hair spray.

By the way, straightened hair reacts to humidity, and it should be protected from salt water and chlorine just as bleached or tinted hair should.

Often it's best to learn to live with your very curly hair. First, I recommend having it cut in a way that follows the natural hair pattern, a length that hits the first arc of the curl on your head. And wear it short. Or let it grow really long and let the weight help overcome the curl. Very frizzy hair should be long enough so that you can control it by pulling it back—and no bangs. Bangs are very hard to control when the hair is quite curly. They will always be a bunch of little squiggles right at the top of your forehead and possibly quite unattractive.

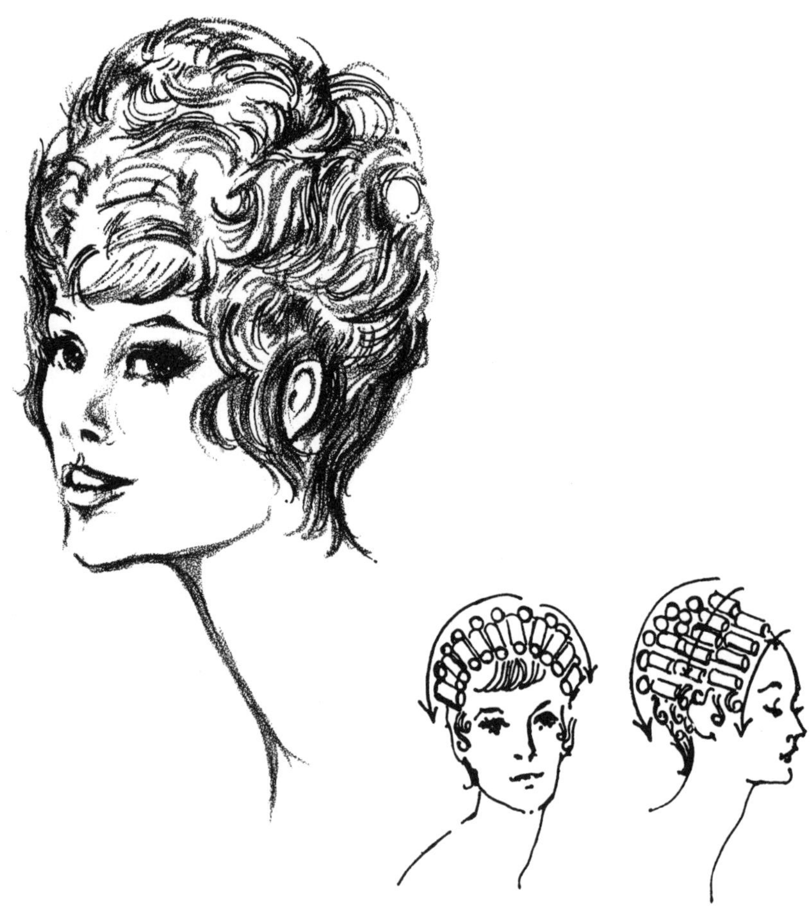

Never allow your hair to be thinned when it is cut because those little short thin ends will curl up and produce a look of terrible bulk. And, as always, I recommend a blunt cut with scissors.

If you don't want to use a hair straightener but wish to have a straighter look, use a heavy cream-type conditioner or rinse (if your texture is not very fine), and a strong setting lotion. Set your hair on very large rollers and make sure the hair is thoroughly dry before you take them out. Try one of the new hold-straight lotions. It may be helpful.

Use a hair dryer instead of letting your hair dry in the air. Somehow heat helps to control frizzing. Or, instead of setting the hair, try using a hot comb or a hand dryer and a brush to stretch the hair and give temporary straightening. A curling iron can be used to pull through the hair and literally iron it straighter. Some people are helped, too, by combing the hair straight down with setting lotion or gel and drying it this way. There is also a "wrap set" which can help control curly hair. (See Chapter 5.)

Frizzy Hair

Some women have hair which isn't really obviously curly or wavy, it's just plain frizzy. And the least bit of humidity will bring out the frizz, even after it's set and smooth.

This frizzy hair is, in reality, curly hair. It's the extreme form of curly hair with a *very* tiny wave pattern. There are many answers to this problem, though none of them really solve it completely.

There is straightening which I advise frizzy-haired people to have done only once a year, preferably just before the hot and humid summer months. At the most, have it done twice a year, but never more than that.

There is the answer of having your hair long enough to be able to pull it straight back in an elastic or barrette and held securely and tightly. Some women even set their hair this way: Shampoo your hair. While it's still wet, apply some strong setting lotion and comb it straight back very slick. Catch it in a covered elastic—while

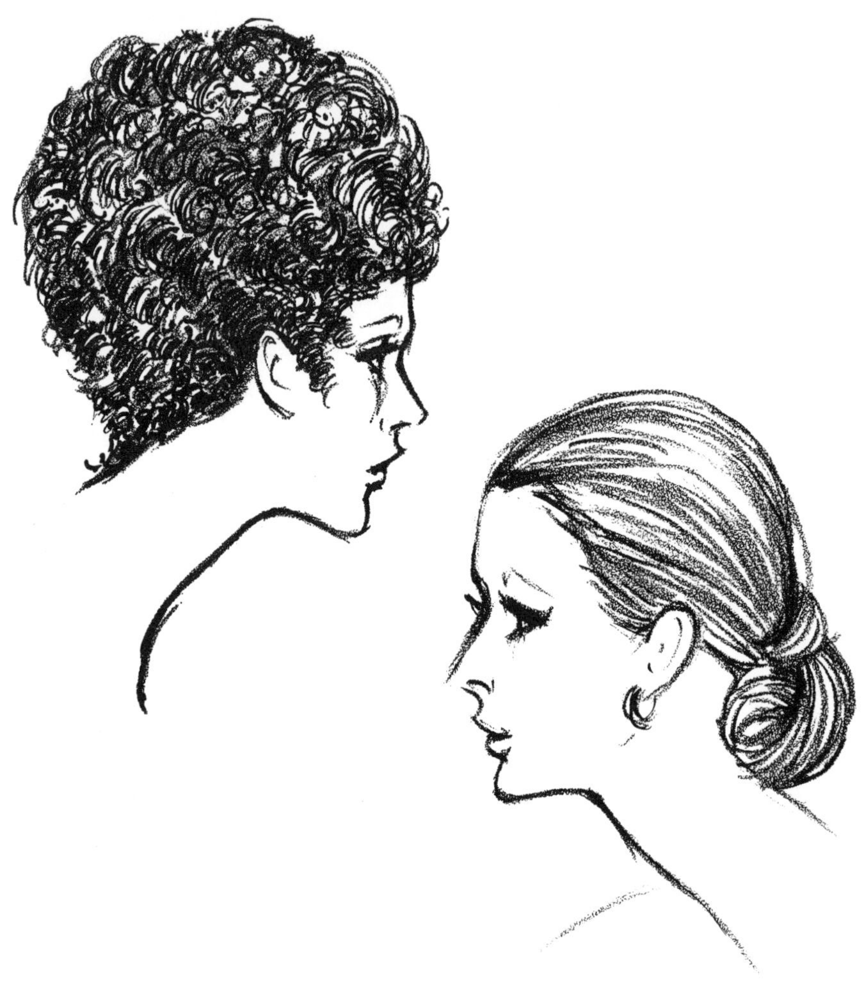

the hair is still soaking wet—and put a couple of big rollers in the ends. Then dry it right in the set.

For some people shorter layered hair works better because the amount of frizziness in their hair does not allow it to stay smooth more than a day after a set. It's easier to set hair every day if it's short.

More and more young women lately frankly admit their hair is frizzy, have it cut into a good shape and leave it *au naturel.* It can look quite enchanting. I realize that if you've grown up thinking that frizzy hair is a curse, this natural style will probably not seem to be the answer for you, but think about it.

If your frizzy hair is coarse and strong, you'll find that cream rinses and cream-based hair conditioners, setting lotions and hold-straight lotions can be temporary aids in smoothing it out. Use the largest size rollers you can get your hair around to make only one turn. Put a fair amount of tension on the rollers to straighten out the wave pattern. If you have *fine* frizzy hair, then avoid the cream preparations because they'll make everything worse. Just try a good firm setting lotion.

A little trick we sometimes use is to spray a piece of cotton with hair spray and gently wipe it on the hairline which will help control the frizziness there without getting a spray build-up on the entire length of hair. Often the frizziness is most bothersome around the face.

Electric combs can help to overcome a certain amount of frizziness. So can electric curlers with the large-size rollers, though I don't suggest their use on a daily basis. You might try blowing your hair dry, smoothing or slightly straightening it with the heat and the air and the brushing. If your hair frizzes up again, spray some water on it just on the top, and blow it dry again to smooth it out.

Your chief concern should be to get a really good haircut, because if your hair has form and shape, even when it begins to go frizzy the crisp shape remains and it doesn't look bad.

Very Coarse Straight Hair

If you have extremely coarse hair that is straight, I don't think you should try to make it curly. It would require all kinds of tapering, thinning, layering, permanenting and other forms of softening. That takes a terrible toll and has a tendency to make the hair dry, brittle and lifeless. Further more, it usually doesn't work.

If the coarser texture of the hair, which sometimes has an almost glassy quality to it, is a problem, it can be most easily helped by

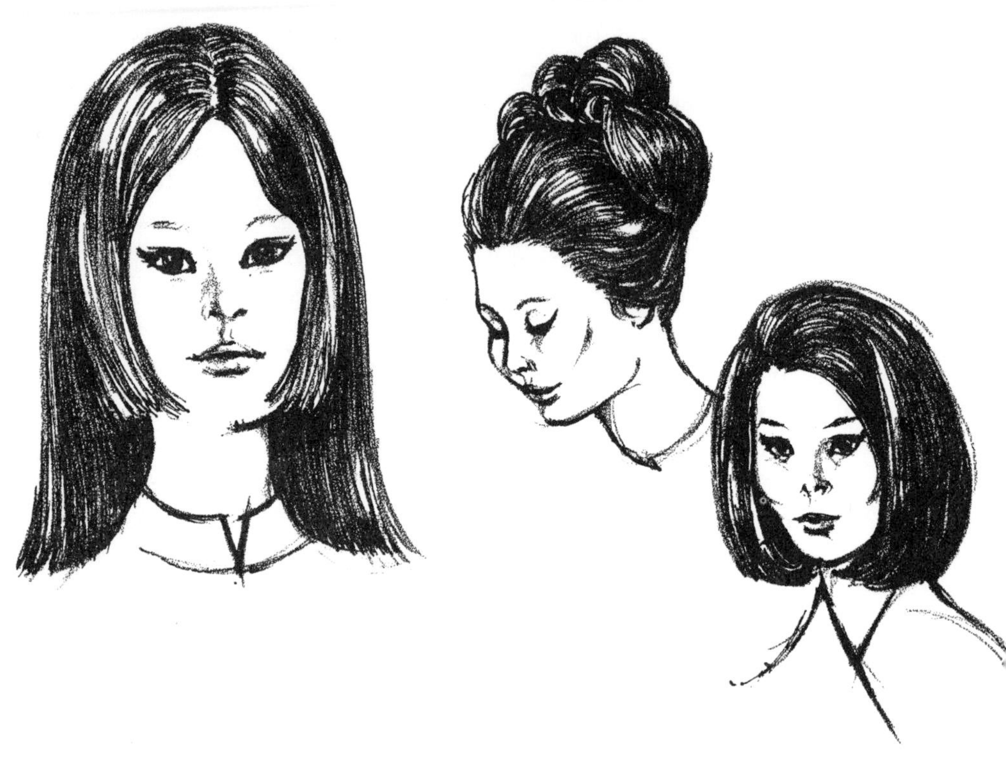

cream rinses, non-alcoholic setting lotion and a softening conditioner.

A simple kind of haircut is best for you, one which allows the hair to swing freely and evenly around the head, either straight or with the ends turned up or under just slightly. And perhaps with bangs, if the direction of the hair at the hairline permits them easily. You could wear this hair pulled up into a chignon or even tied back at the nape of the neck.

It will be helpful if your hair is cut with the top layer a bit longer, to encourage it to curl under. Usually a longer style works better than a short one for you.

One thing that can be helpful with your kind of hair is a body wave on the most enormous permanent-wave rods, one-half inch to one inch in diameter. This is really a kind of softening action rather than a waving action. In a sense, it breaks down the natural stiffness of the hair. And what you are always looking for is something to make the hair softer and more pliable.

If your hair is dry as well as stiff a finishing hairdressing cream may be a help too.

Dry Hair

Is dry hair your problem? I hear complaints about it every day of my life and it's understandable because dry hair is usually dull and lifeless and never looks smooth. It's hard to curl. It tends to fly about and have a lot of static electricity, all because the scalp does not produce sufficient natural oil.

The dryness can be your normal scalp condition, or it may have been caused by the excessive use of chemicals on your hair and scalp—such as coloring, straightening, permanenting, etc.

You are the perfect customer for one of those conditioners that is designed to lubricate the hair. Use an instant conditioner every time you shampoo your hair—which shouldn't be too often—and a longer conditioning treatment about once a month.

Never wash your hair more often than once a week and try to let it go a day or so longer. Unless you live in a highly air-polluted community, it won't need it as dry hair doesn't attract dirt the way oily hair does.

Choose a shampoo designed especially for dry hair. We use an egg-and-oil formula at my salon.

An old-fashioned but good remedy for your situation, if it's your *scalp* that's dry and not merely the ends of the hair, is to warm some castor oil (or olive, mineral, salad, etc.) and massage it into the scalp before you wash it. Wrap your head in hot steamy towels for fifteen minutes and then wash. Or wrap it in a dry towel and sit under a dryer set at "low" for ten minutes. NOTE: Castor oil is very hard to get out of the hair. You'll need hot water and some good sudsings. (See "Hot-Oil Treatments" in Chapter 3.)

If the ends of your hair are dry, but not your scalp, you can apply the oil only to the ends and leave it on for ten or fifteen minutes before shampooing.

To encourage the flow of oils from the scalp, I'd suggest a good brushing and a vigorous scalp massage every day.

I've known several people with very dry scalp and hair who have taken up yoga and found the condition of their hair has changed since they learned to stand on their heads. You really *can* learn to stand on your head—you should see some of the people I know who can—but if you'd rather not, spend some time every day with your head lower than the trunk of your body, either on a slant board or by bending over or lying over the edge of the bed so you get more circulation in your head.

Never dry your hair with very high heat. If you have the time, it would be best to use no heat at all but rather dry it in the air.

Avoid the chemical processes such as overbleaching, permanenting and straightening, which are harsh and drying. Even coloring can be drying. Stay away from hair sprays containing excessive lacquer. People with extremely dry hair must cover it when they're out in the sun if they don't want it to turn to straw, and should immediately rinse or wash out salt water or chlorinated pool water. But then, so should everybody else!

Damaged Hair

Most hair starts out happy and healthy. But often it's then ruined by too much of everything—too much bleaching, dyeing, spraying, sunning, straightening, permanenting, etc. Perhaps a straightener was left on too long and the hair is breaking off. Perhaps you've had an overprocessed permanent or one that was wound too tightly. Maybe your hair has been damaged by excessive coloring or bleaching, where the chemicals were applied to the same hair over and over, rather than just to the new hair at the roots. It is astounding to me that people do such extraordinary things to their hair under the guise of fashion. They end up with hair that's no longer hair, no longer a beautiful fabric. It's so sad that people get themselves in such terrible shape by not using common sense. The damage that's done is irreparable, and there's no way to overcome it.

I know a model who had the most beautiful hair I'd ever seen. I didn't see her for six or eight months, and then she came in for a setting before a photographic session. Her hair had been ruined; it was split, all different lengths, dry and brittle. I said, "My god, what have you done to your hair?" She'd been straightening and coloring her hair, then using heated curlers twice a day every day for months. The constant handling had done the dirty work. And now nothing can repair her hair until it grows out.

That is the point. Once your hair is damaged, you cannot cure it. You must wait until it all grows out and once again you have shiny, soft, healthy, natural hair.

It is possible, however, to give damaged hair some protection and make it look better until it is replaced by nature. Here the conditioners can be helpful. Most of them involve ingredients that act as fillers for the hair shaft or as coatings, smoothing them out or making them seem thicker.

Some hair-conditioning specialists will give you special treatments which may include ultraviolet light and heat caps and maybe steroid lotion. These specialists are not easy to find, however, outside of the largest cities, so you'll probably have to cope with your damaged hair yourself.

If your hair is particularly limp and bodiless you might try one of the texturizers or bodybuilders now on the market. These are essentially fillers and often work very well the first few times you use them. I've found, though, that they tend to dry out the hair, so I suggest using them for a couple of weeks and then stopping for a while.

The basic approach to damaged hair is to leave it alone. Wear it in as becoming a style as possible, preferably short because then you will be constantly cutting off much of the bad hair. A style that might get you past a damaged head of hair is a very short cut like the illustration on the next page, if you can wear it. Then let it grow out without putting any more stress and strain on it. Don't tint it, don't bleach it, don't permanent or straighten it. Leave it alone. If it looks really terrible, buy a couple of wigs and wear them until your own hair is bearable.

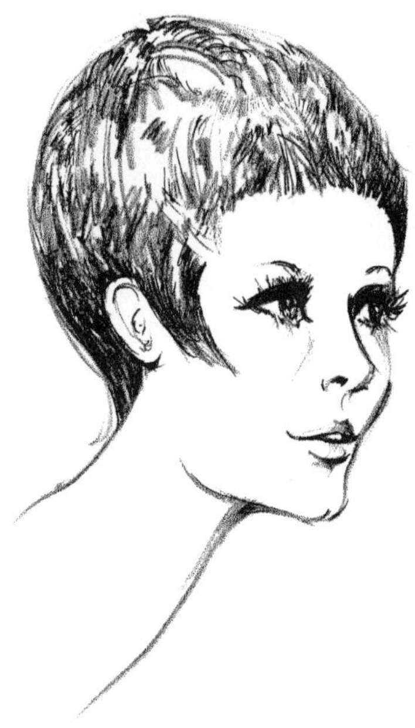

Keep your hair clean by washing with a gentle shampoo, and use the conditioner each time. Give it daily but gentle brushing, bending over so that your head is lower than the rest of you. Don't brush too much or too hard because that way you may break the weakened hair. A gentle scalp massage every day can be helpful in getting the oil glands stimulated.

And when your new hair grows out again, take better care of it this time!

Slow-Growing Hair

Hair grows on an average of one-half inch per month and, while I've been told that God made us all equal, there are exceptions to everything. I have known people whose hair grows as much as an inch a month and others whose hair seems to grow much more slowly than a half inch a month. Either way, there's nothing you can do about it. Most important, you must keep the ends of your hair trimmed, even if you're trying to grow it, to discourage breaking and splitting. People think trimming makes the hair grow faster. It doesn't. It just seems that way because it's not breaking off at the ends.

There is no way to make your hair grow faster, though the rate does change at different times of the year and speeds up a bit in hot weather. And some people's hair will never grow very long. Most hairs last for three to five years. If your hair grows faster than average and lasts longer than average, you will be able to grow very long hair. But if it grows slowly and is replaced in only three years or so, it will never grow very, very long.

Split Ends

These are usually the result of damage or daily wear and tear and make the hair look dry and lighter colored at the ends. They come from too much bleaching, straightening, curling, permanenting, too constant use of heated curlers, brush rollers, too much sun and chlorine and all the other miserable tortures you can submit your hair to. Stop!!

Once you've got split ends, the only thing you can do about them is to have them trimmed off regularly, about every four weeks. This is important because the longer a split remains, the farther it travels up the hair shaft.

Don't continue the foolish belief in magic potions to cure split ends. Keep your hair trimmed properly, and split ends will almost disappear.

Dandruff

Nobody knows what causes dandruff, but everybody knows what a terrible nuisance it is. It's a common affliction and hopefully there will soon be a way to do away with it. Dandruff is excessive scaling of the scalp, sometimes itchy and always unattractive. If your head is dry, the dandruff flakes off your scalp freely and falls on your shoulders. If your head is oily, the scales stick together and come off in larger pieces. It can spread to your eyebrows or behind your ears. Either way, it's hateful.

It is possible to think you have dandruff when you really don't. Everyone's head sheds dead skin cells and that little bit of flaking that appears sometimes is not necessarily dandruff. I've known people whose heads have been sunburned and then peeled, and they thought they had dandruff. Sometimes women don't rinse the soap out of their hair well enough or they use a hair spray that flakes when it's brushed out. That isn't dandruff either.

Occasionally people notice the appearance of dandruff—real dandruff—during a tense time in their lives. And sometimes it's when they are terribly tired. If dandruff appears suddenly and dramatically, a visit to the doctor is a good idea as it is whenever there is an abrupt change in your physical condition. It may signify a more general problem. And if your case seems especially severe, maybe with bleeding or oozing, you should certainly check with him. He may prescribe steroid lotion or ultraviolet light or even injections.

But so far as I have ever heard, no cure has been found for real, honest, persistent dandruff. There are, however, some ways to control it to a certain extent. The first basic approach to dandruff is to wash your hair often, whenever the dandruff begins to be noticeable. Use a shampoo especially designed to control dandruff—it will definitely help. Try the various brands until you find the one which works best for you; one will probably work better on your particular variety of dandruff than another. I've also found that people build up a tolerance to things—a shampoo will work for them for a long time and then it won't. If you switch for a while, it will help. Always be sure to do an extraordinary amount of rinsing after a shampoo, ending with cool running water for a few minutes.

I suggest you give yourself a scalp massage every day or at least before every shampoo. This will help keep the scalp loose and get the circulation going, and is especially helpful if your scalp is dry. It will also loosen up the scales and make them easier to brush or wash out. When you massage, be very gentle, being careful never to scratch or irritate the scalp. It's important, too, never to use a brush with sharp bristles. Dandruff is bad enough without having a secondary infection along with it.

Because emotional stress and a faulty diet are thought to have some connection with dandruff, it's obviously best to get enough sleep and relaxation, and to eat well-balanced meals.

Dull Hair

Some hair is just plain dull. It has no life, no sparkle, no brightness, no shine. There are shades of ash blond which have a tendency to absorb light rather than reflect it. Some pale browns have a dead look. Textures make a difference too. Coarse hair tends to be shinier or brighter than fine hair which may, especially if you have a lot of it, pack down and get a solid look to it.

The only real solution for naturally dull hair is to add highlights to it by streaking or shading. Perhaps some red highlights or blond streaking will do it. Sometimes just lightening the area around the hairline or on top of the head will make an enormous difference. Or, of course, you can change the color of the entire head.

Occasionally dull hair comes from not rinsing all the soap out after a shampoo. I know that the water is extremely hard in many parts of the country, and even though you add water softeners, the soap can be hard to rinse out. You can buy a special soap-curd remover and use it in the last rinse. Or try the home remedy of mixing a tablespoon of borax into a gallon of water and rinsing with that.

Excessively dry hair that splits a lot will often look dull, and the use of a good conditioner can help.

A more common cause of dullness is excessive tinting. The problem is that the hair becomes one color all over the head. By nature, nobody's hair is all one color. I suggest you have your hair colored —by a professional—in variegated shadings or tone-on-tone. Or make the hairline slightly lighter, or perhaps streak the hair two shades lighter all over, to give a brighter look.

If you've been tinting your hair for a long time, you may have a build-up of coloring on the hair which will cause it to look lifeless. An occasional hot-oil treatment given by a professional will take away some of that excess coating.

There are pomades and hair-finishing creams to be rubbed on the hand and skimmed over the hair to give a sheen. You might try these if your hair is dry, or one of the spray-on products designed to add glinty highlights might do it for you. They'll work until they wear off.

Pregnancy and Your Hair

Most women have no more trouble with their hair when pregnant than at any other time. But some find it becomes quite limp, maybe oily, and soils quickly because of increased scalp perspiration. If this happens to you, you'll just have to live with it, knowing there's a cure at the end of the nine months. I'd suggest a shortish simple wash-and-wear haircut, or hair long enough to pull back in some contained way. The virtue of both of these, too, is that when you are in the hospital your hair will look good even though you obviously can't have it set.

Wash your hair as often as it needs it to remove the oil and the perspiration. Keep it well groomed. During pregnancy, there is usually little or no normal hair loss so that you'll end up with thicker hair than you had before. But after the childbirth, it may thin out markedly. In most cases, the loss isn't extreme and the hair returns to normal in several months. Occasionally, though, it remains thin and I suggest asking a dermatologist for possible remedies.

Chapter 5

CUTS AND SETS

Cutting

Hair is beautiful, it seems to me, if it is free and natural, something you want to run your fingers through. And that's the hardest hair to achieve because it depends on a good, a really good, haircut. Properly cut hair is the answer to most people's hair problems. And it isn't easy to get.

There are too few hairdressers who know how to cut hair. A good haircut, to my mind, can only be achieved with scissors. Clients tell

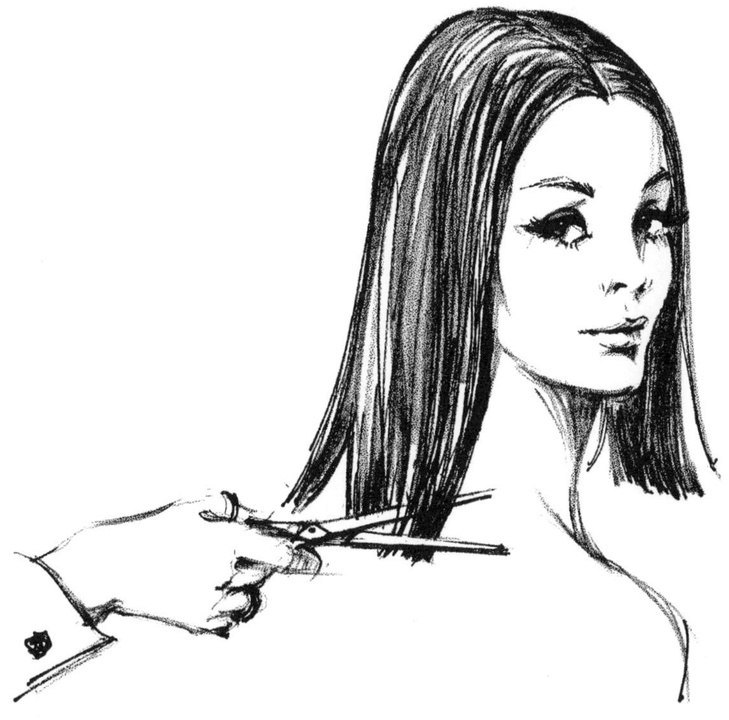

me constantly that some hairdressers say this is nonsense, that they can give them a good cut with a razor. I say, "The next time they tell you that, get right up out of the chair and leave." A razor will always taper or slither or thin the ends of the hair as it's cut, thus reducing its natural body. A scissors always produces the same thickness at the end of the hair as it has at the base, thereby retaining whatever the natural body your hair may have. Cutting with scissors produces a "blunt" cut which means cutting straight across each hair.

This does *not* mean that you must have hair that is all one length. Your hair may be blunt-cut into a layered style as well. "Layering" means just that—cutting the hair in layers of equal length all over the head.

Hairdressers use razors because they think that the hair will be easier to tease and to curl. I see women all over the country with their hair thinned or slithered at the ends by razors—or, sometimes, even with scissors—because someone advised them the curl would hold better that way. But it doesn't, and when their hair comes out of the set, I don't know what these women have except shapelessness. Nothing is left and they look terrible. With a good blunt cut, you can have a good basic shape, wet or dry. What you do with it depends on the setting. You don't change the cut, merely the set. I am against trying to force the hair to do something it's simply not made to do.

Each hairdresser goes about giving you a haircut in his own way. The method isn't really important. I myself go through the hair section by section and I know that when I end up every hair will fall into the shape I'm after. You should judge the haircut not only by its finished look and the way it behaves, but by the length of time it takes. I can't believe a good haircut can be done in less than twenty minutes at the very least. There just aren't any short cuts.

I always cut the hair wet, after it's been shampooed, because there is no old set to battle with. The hair comes down to its longest length, and when you comb it through, it doesn't fly all over the place. I can also see its natural wave, if any; or how much permanent is left. I really see what the hair is like. Another important point in seeing a client first with her hair wet is that my vision of her looks is not colored by the hairdo she has had. I don't want to know how she was wearing her hair. I want to get my own ideas.

I part the hair so that I can work in sections, one by one. Otherwise I would be just picking hair up out of the blue. To get the right length, I always pin up the top layers and cut the back underneath first. The hair at the nape always establishes the shape and the allover length that the haircut is ultimately going to have. It's the only logical place to start cutting.

Then I bring down the rest, a section at a time. If I want it all one length, but longer in the front, I can establish this when I am matching the side sections to the back by cutting them at an angle that runs longer toward the face. The desirability of this kind of shape, in a modified form, is that when the hair is combed back from the hairline it will all hang absolutely evenly around the head. This is especially good for young people.

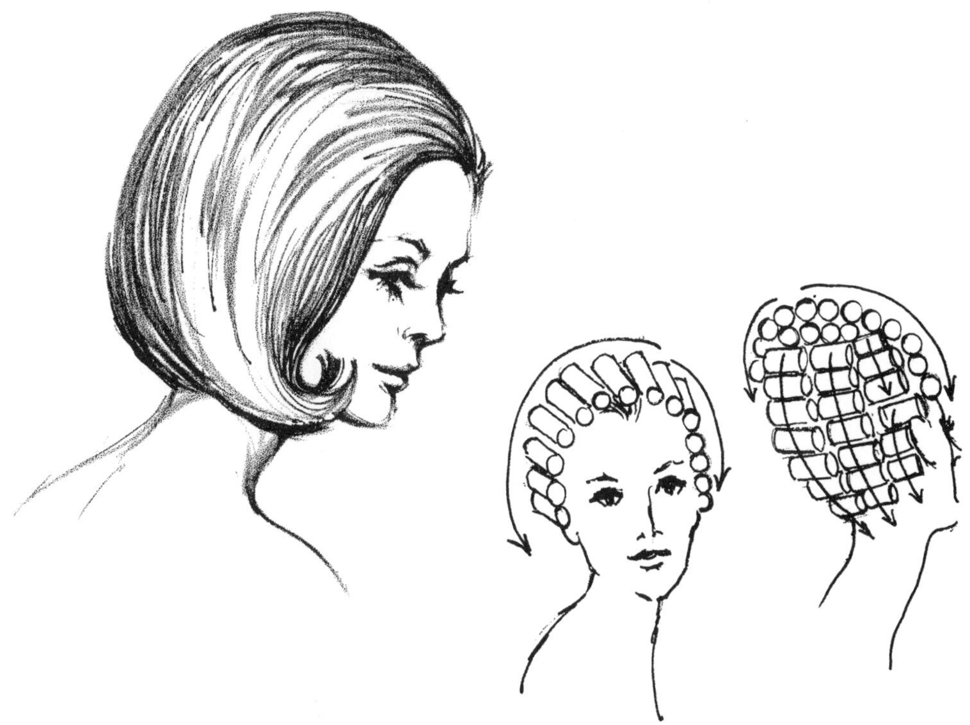

Many people find, however, that the extra length in front is hard to keep back from the face and consequently unflattering to them if they are not so young. Therefore, we often cut the hair absolutely even all one length around the head, and sometimes gradually shorter toward the face. But it is still all-one-length hair. In other words, there is no layering.

If it's to be a layered cut the basic change is that, after I have established the length the hair will be after cutting the first one or two sections at the nape, I do *not* bring the next section down and cut it to match the bottom length. I hold the hair straight out from the head and cut as the bottom hair drops away. This means that what I am actually doing is cutting each hair the same length all

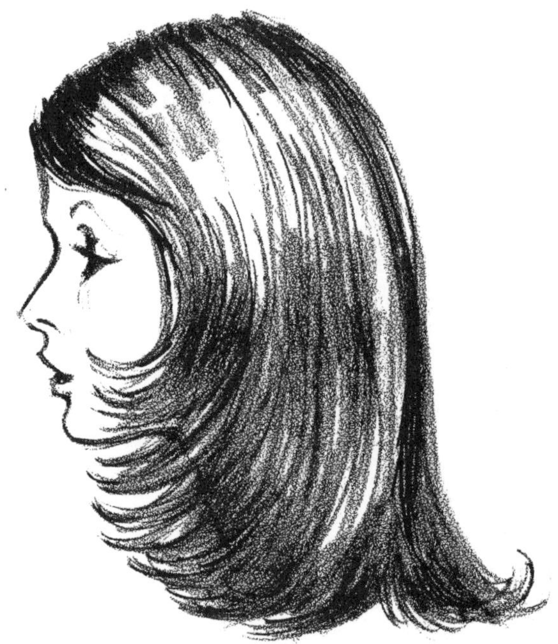

over the head. If the hair at the nape is three inches long the hair at the crown is three inches long, and the hair at the front is three inches long. This is, of course, a very basic way of explaining a layered haircut. There are many variations. In a good layered cut, you don't see each layer—it all blends together.

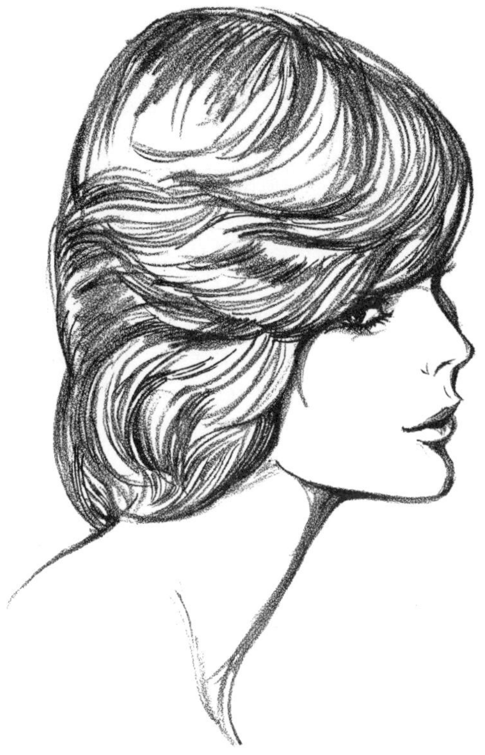

It takes me a long time to do a cut—that's why it's so expensive. Clients pay for my expertise, my reputation and my time.

Never allow a hairdresser to thin your hair. Never. You can cut, shape, layer, give any kind of style or line to a head of hair *without thinning*. I am dead against it. Nobody has ever been able to prove to me that thinning does not remove the hair's natural body. And body is what we look for today. Body is bulk, thickness, weight. In other words, luxurious hair.

The women who usually insist on thinning are the ones who have very thick, curly or frizzy hair. Thinning will only make this kind of hair behave even worse. It will produce little short ends all over the head which, especially in damp weather, will stand up and look frizzier. A good hair stylist can cut your hair in a much more manageable shape without the thinning scissors.

Setting

I think we'll find in the next ten years that hair setting, as we've known it, will be done less and less. There will be more settings done just with a hand-held hair dryer, or hot combs, or merely placing the hair and sitting under a dryer. If your hair is set this way, you'll probably have to wash it more often than you did when it was done via the more familiar roller set, maybe every day. But it only takes about ten minutes, and if you'd like a little volume somewhere, say, on the crown, you can achieve that with a curling iron or a couple of heated rollers. To set your hair this way, you must have an excellent haircut—that is absolutely essential. You get a good haircut and then you do the setting yourself.

You'd think that a hairdresser would recommend that every woman go to a beauty salon to have her hair done every week, rather than show her how to do the job at home. But, aside from the women who have the new non-set hair styles, there are more and more people today who go to a hairdresser only when they need a haircut and who prefer to do their own conventional settings. Besides, many clients, who may be salon regulars, want to know how to set their own hair, especially in the summer when it needs more washing, or they are away from their regular hairdresser. Women with oily hair, particularly, can't always wait to get to the salon.

I believe every hairdo, except for the more elaborate evening arrangements, should be possible to reproduce at home. It does take practice to set hair properly and especially to comb it so it will look good and stay put for a while. But there is nothing strange or magical about it. You can learn to do a good job yourself, once you've got a good cut and styling. Ask your hairdresser how the rollers should be placed for the style you've been wearing—I'm sure he will even provide you with a little sketch of the pattern—and what size rollers to use. Or ask for a lesson in blowing dry your hair or "placing" it. Be willing to pay for the lesson. It's worth it if it will give you good-looking hair on a daily basis.

In order to set your hair well, you must understand why you are doing it because you get out of a set exactly what you put into it. The purpose of setting the hair is to tell a good haircut what to do when it's dry. It gives added body or curl or wave or straightness to the shape and form you have. It makes the best of it. Any set must direct the hair into the line in which it grows or in which it's been cut. If the set fights with your hair, it won't last longer than a half hour unless it's sprayed into concrete. For years now, the general practice has been to set hair with almost no direction and then spend a half hour combing it out and forcing it into a shape or a line. That is wrong. If the set is good, the combing will be easy.

When you set your hair, you are giving it temporary curl or direction. The diameter of the roller or pin curl determines the amount of curl you'll get. Rollers and stand-up pin curls will give you a full curl. Flat pin curls will give you a close, tight head or deep waves. Blowing dry will produce volume and a small amount of bend. Place sets will be flat.

After you've shampooed your hair, towel-dry it, then brush it even drier. If your hair is very fine and bodiless, it will take a firmer set if you dry it completely after the shampoo so that you'll get the benefit of the full strength of the setting lotion.

Now apply the setting lotion. There are lotions, gels, creams and sprays, and all of them work well if you use them correctly. Follow the directions on the package. It's necessary for a good set that the lotion totally covers the entire hair shaft of every hair you are curling. Your set will not be good if some hair is wet and some hair is dry. That is why the thinner lotions are easier for most people to cope with. But if you prefer a cream or gel because it has a firmer action on your hair, I have no objection if you comb it through the hair thoroughly and evenly.

A problem you'll run into if you choose a lotion or gel which gives extra firm body to the hair is that you may also discover your hair won't be as bouncy and shiny as you'd like, and that you'll have to shampoo it more often.

Make the hair very wet with the lotion. I always soak it until it's dripping. Obviously, you will need a towel around your shoulders if you do that. And I personally prefer to use a spray-on lotion because it provides more uniform coverage.

I like to spray liquid setting lotion over the hair again *after* it's rolled up because then you are spraying the base or the roots of the hair which may not have been thoroughly saturated before. This is the place where you need to get as much body as you can; that's where you get the lift.

There are a few different kinds of sets—roller, pin curl, blow-dry, wrap set, place set, to name some.

Rollers

Rollers are the most popular way of setting hair because they give it lift and volume—they're really pin curls standing up. The first thing to remember is that the smaller the rollers, the tighter the curl or the wave pattern you will produce. The size of the rollers controls the amount of body you will get too. Generally, the coarser your hair, the larger the rollers you'll need; the finer your hair, the smaller you'll need. It's illogical for a girl with very fine hair to set her hair on very big rollers and expect the set is going to last.

Sizes of rollers range from a half inch to three inches in diameter, and they come in many types. Never, never use the brush rollers, as they are harmful both to the hair and to the scalp. They catch onto the hair and hold it, causing breakage and tangling. And the sharp bristles irritate the scalp.

Smooth plastic or metal rollers are fine, but they are hard to work with as they slip too easily. I prefer the plastic or wire mesh rollers which wind easily and allow air to circulate through the hair, drying it more quickly and evenly.

To keep the ends smooth and prevent them from frizzing, I like using end papers. The papers also make the rolling easier because they contain all the little wisps of hair in one compact package.

And I prefer clips to bobby pins for holding the rollers in place, as they don't make the ridges that bobby pins make on the hair. Be sure the clips are snug. They do loosen up after a lot of use. If yours do, throw them out and invest in some new ones.

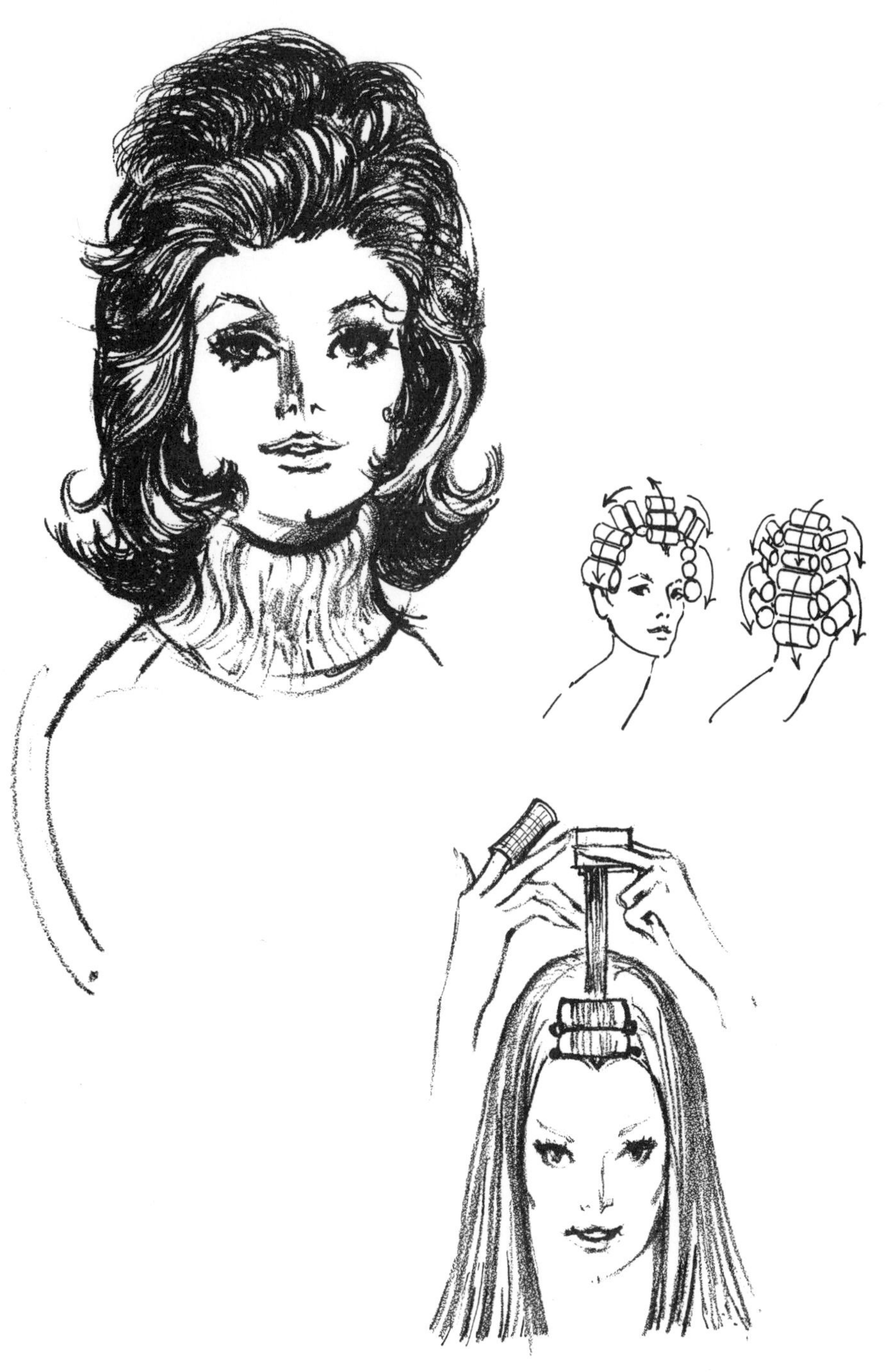

After you have thoroughly wet your hair with setting lotion, section off a piece of hair which is about an inch deep and a half inch narrower than the roller—the wet hair will spread as it is rolled and dried. Comb the hair straight up from the scalp; hold it there with your fingers. For more height, stretch the hair in the *opposite* direction from which it's to be rolled. This is to make sure the hair right from the scalp is curled, that there's no long stem before it starts to curl.

Now fold an end paper over the hair, slide it to the ends and hold firmly. Place the roller next to the end paper and, keeping the hair quite taut and spread out, never bunched all together in the middle, slowly roll down to the scalp. The tension is most important. The hair must be wound smoothly, tautly and evenly, but never really pulled so it lifts the scalp up with it. This is unhealthy and unnecessary and usually happens because the winding at the ends is sloppy and so the roller is made tighter as it's wound down to the scalp.

Attach the first roller with clips—at its base. Never place the clip at the top of the roller because it will leave marks on the finished hairdo. Then attach the next roller to the first one, the third one to the second one and so on.

Pin Curls

Flat pin curls are best when you want a close-to-the-head style because they don't produce as much lift as rollers. Or they're good when the hair is too short for rollers, or if you want a pickup dry set. Often they're used in combination with rollers, usually at the cheeks or in the back where the hair is short, or where you want flat or soft curls. Flat pin curls give a flatter turn to the hair. To give hair more volume, make stand-up pin curls.

Again, the smaller the pin curls, the tighter the curl or wave pattern.

To make pin curls, pick up a small section of wet hair, no bigger than a half inch in diameter. Hold it straight up with your thumb

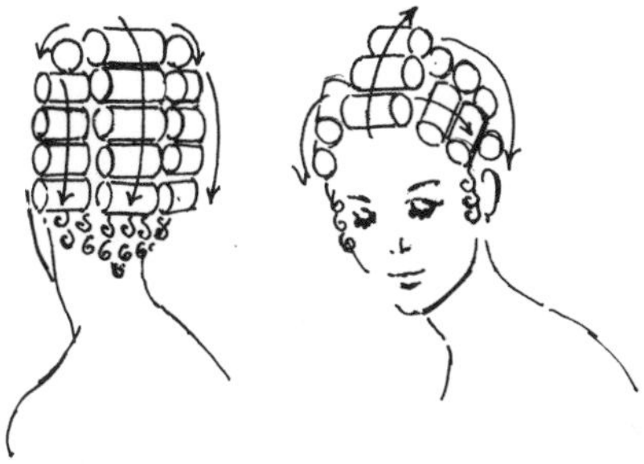

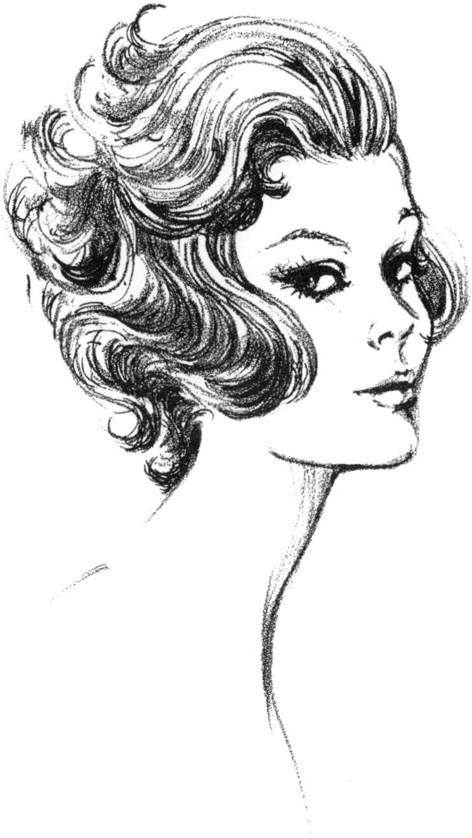

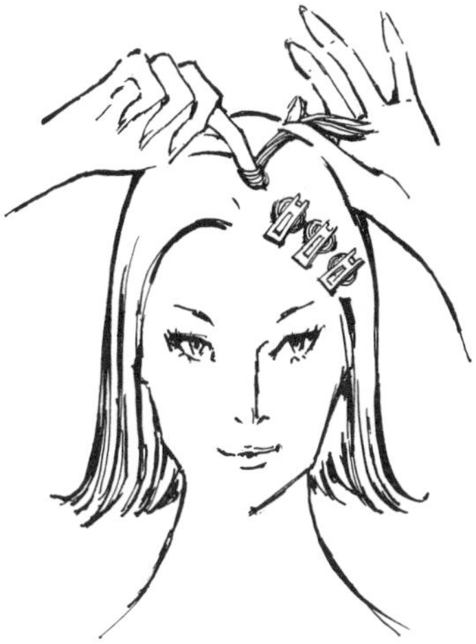

and forefinger. Now start curling it with your fingers right at the scalp, so that it immediately has direction and all of the hair has movement. Continue to curl the strand, making sure that the curl

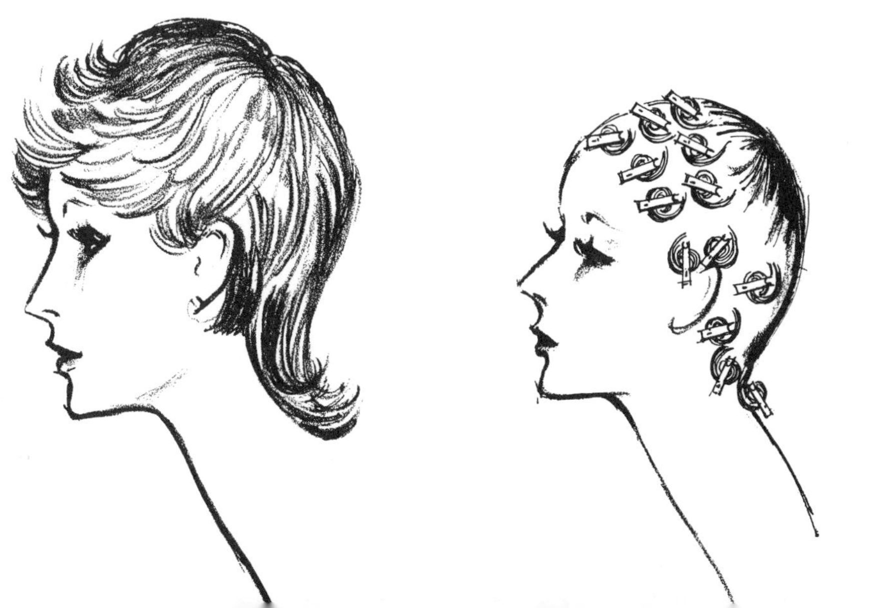

remains the same circumference all the way to the ends. If it gets smaller and smaller, it will come out kinked and uneven.

Start making the pin curls at the top of the head, then on the sides, then at the back and nape.

Secure the pin curls with a clip or a bobby pin. I prefer clips because they leave less of a mark on the hair and are easier to slip on. Always fasten the clip with the points *toward the stem* of the curl as it will be less likely to make ridges or to affect the shape of the curls. To make a stand-up curl, clip only through the outer half of it, leaving the stem half free.

Bangs

For bouncy bangs, set on rollers or over cotton. If you want them flat, however, comb them straight down with setting lotion and hold with clips or a ribbon around your head. Or just let them dry in place.

Drying

Allow the hair to dry thoroughly and evenly, either under a dryer or in the air, testing to make sure it isn't still damp before you remove the rollers or pin curls. Remove rollers gently, carefully unwinding each one to the very end of the strand before pulling it out. Be sure the ends are dry. And, while I'm on the subject, may I ask that you don't wear rollers or pin curls out in public? I remember one Saturday evening when I was out of town on a working trip. I went to a local theater production and sitting in the front row was a woman with all her hair in rollers. I figured that woman must never be out of those rollers. If going out on Saturday night isn't going out, what is?

And I'm sure your husband finds rollers in bed just as revolting as they seem to me. Hair eternally in rollers is not just ugly but it is unhealthy, putting great strain on the hair and scalp and preventing free circulation of air. When you sleep on rollers, you'll not only be mighty uncomfortable, but will be tugging dangerously on your hair, producing hair loss, breakage and loss of elasticity. While drying your hair with a dryer may take some of the natural oils out, it may, on the other hand, be preferable to spending your life in rollers.

Brush-out

The purpose of combing is to place the hair where it belongs, putting it back into the shape it was cut to, though perhaps curlier, wavier, straighter or smoother. It is not difficult to do a good comb-out if the haircut is good and the setting is organized.

I always brush out a set totally. People are often afraid to brush their hair, afraid they'll take out the set. But if it's a good set the brushing makes it better, gets it all together, erases the roller separations.

If the hair is stiff with setting lotion, comb through each curl individually to loosen the stiffness. If you brush right through rigid sets you can easily break the hair.

Always brush the hair thoroughly from front to back, no matter what the style will be, so that the curl is evenly distributed, and turn the hair under as if you were going to make a page boy. Then very lightly brush the top layer of hair in the direction you've set it until you get the shape you want. Now that you have the shape, take a hairpin (you can use a rattail comb, if you like) and loosen the hair underneath very gently, pulling out pieces here and there until the form is right.

For curly hairdos which are to look free and natural, it's a good idea to use your fingers to pull the hair around after you've finished combing it.

On longer hair where you want to get a look of thickness and volume, this is a good trick: Bend over with your head down. Brush your hair up. Now toss your head back and brush lightly over the top of the hair.

Teasing

Teasing, or back-combing, should not be used the way it usually is. It should not make your hair into a big snarl that's smoothed over on top. It should not build it into a fancy concoction, high and unnatural and stiff. In a funny way, excessive teasing takes *out* your set, which you then reset with hair spray. I just don't want to get involved with the concrete hairdo and I cannot accept that as a way of life for hair. Therefore I say: Tease very lightly or forget about it altogether.

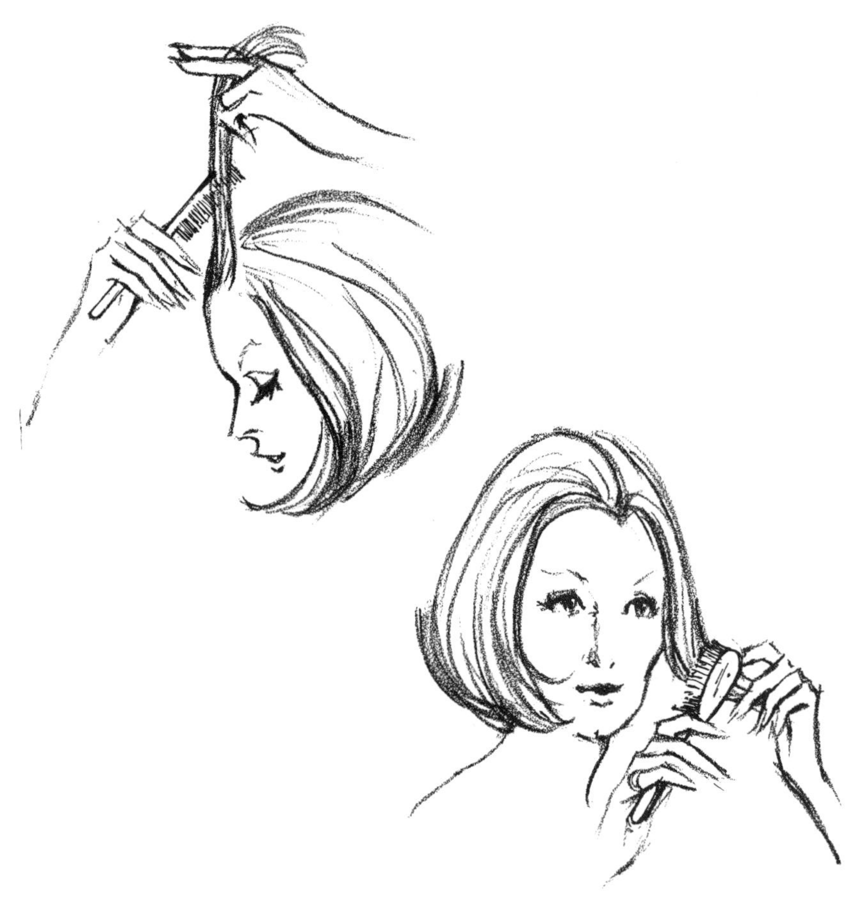

Teasing should be done sparingly. The purpose should be to keep the hair together and to give a certain lift or form in specific spots. My method is very gentle; it goes in with a few swipes of the comb and comes out with a few swipes of the comb. Here's how to do it:

Use a fine comb, not a brush. I feel that teasing with a brush, although it's faster and easier, can cause damage by snarling and breaking the hair. You can't feel what you are doing with a brush. You can be much more controlled using a comb.

Hold a small section of hair straight up from your head with your fingers. Slowly comb the hair from underneath and toward the scalp, using long, even strokes. Start about two inches from the scalp and work slowly toward the ends, combing straight down with each stroke. Do this section by section wherever you need some volume. Now use this fluffed-up hair as a cushion over which you gently brush the top layer of hair. To be even safer, I like to tease only the center of a strand, from the middle down, without touching the ends.

This mild teasing will probably not harm your hair, though continuous, excessive teasing is certainly bad for it.

Probably the most harm is done by combing *out* heavy teasing. Never just yank a brush through it. Start at the ends of the hair, as you should with any tangled hair, brushing until smooth, then work gently toward the scalp. If you start at the base next to the scalp and pull hard, that's when you'll break the hair. Of course, the hair should never be teased so much that it presents a real problem. The only acceptable teasing today is put in with a very light touch.

Always brush teasing out at night—don't sleep on it.

Hair Spray

The lacquered, stiff, glued-together look of hair is outdated. Spray should not be used as a substitute for a haircut or a set or a permanent wave. It should merely be a finish to keep little wispy hairs from flying around.

Try different brands of spray until you find one that doesn't glue your hair together and doesn't dull it either. There are some good ones on the market. Buy small cans till you find yours. After that, the big thing is not to use too much. Hold the can at least ten inches from your head so that only a gentle mist falls on it after it's been combed into shape. Don't saturate it.

Always try to choose an unscented hair spray or one that isn't heavily perfumed. You don't want to smell like hair spray, nor do you want it to interfere with your perfume.

You can use hair spray when you need a touch-up set. Dry-set the hair and then spray it lightly. Let it stay for a half hour or so and then brush out.

Or use hair spray to hold up those little ends of hair that droop down from an upswept hairdo. Comb the hair in place, then take a piece of cotton and spray it. Brush the little ends up with the wet cotton. This is better than spraying the hair because it concentrates the solution just where you need it.

Place Sets

If you have rather short, naturally wavy hair or a really good wash-and-wear haircut, combined with a good texture, you can merely "place" your sopping hair in the shape you want it, and let it dry. First towel-dry the hair after it's shampooed, then comb it into the proper shape, holding it here and there with clips, if necessary, and letting it dry. Make a couple of pin curls, perhaps at the sides, if you need them.

Blow-Dry Sets

This is the newest way to set hair and it's the way more and more women will be using as we get away from the immobile hairdos and into the natural, flowing, bouncy styles of the future. It is perfect for women who are tired of rollers and bobby pins, and will give a

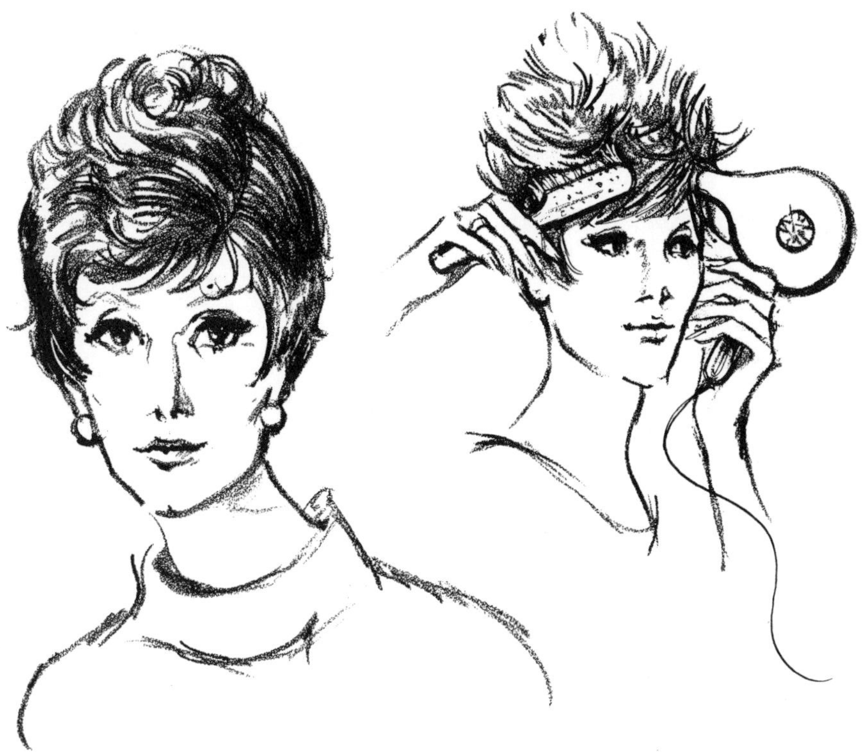

much softer, more natural, less coiffured look. Basically, a blow-dry set is a good haircut which becomes a hair style with the help of a hand dryer and a brush. You blow the hair with hot air and brush it up and around the brush at the same time. The heat and the air of the dryer give a certain volume to the hair and can be used to straighten or smooth it, stretching out a natural wave; or it can be used to dry your natural wave into place. You can give long, straight hair volume this way, as many young girls do, but the blow-dry set is usually associated with rather short hair styles.

Blowing your hair dry seems very simple and it is. However, you do have to know what you're doing if you don't want to end up with just plain flyaway, nowhere hair.

First, I have to insist again, you need a super haircut. This is essential. Without it, you cannot get a good shape, especially if you don't set it in a conventional way. Go to the very best hairdresser you know. Don't try to save money here. Have the hairdresser give you a blow-dry set and watch how he does it so you can do it yourself at home.

To blow-dry your super haircut, towel-dry it first. Then fluff it up a bit with your fingers to dry it even more. Comb it out with a wide-toothed comb until every tangle is gone and the hair lies flat on your head. I usually recommend that you don't apply any setting lotion, though a *little* spray may be helpful later if, as it dries, your hair has tremendous static electricity.

Blow-dry sets are done with a rounded brush and a small lightweight hand dryer, which should have a lot of heat and air power as these are what give the hair body and shape.

If your haircut is up to, say, three inches long all over your head you can probably do the drying only with the dryer and your fingers. Blow it in the direction the style will be worn when it's finished.

If the hair is longer than three inches chances are a brush or comb and a hand dryer are what you'll need. You brush the hair and stretch and form it while it is blowing dry. This will produce a hair style which is close to the head and it works best on hair that is naturally fairly straight. Pick up a section of hair with the

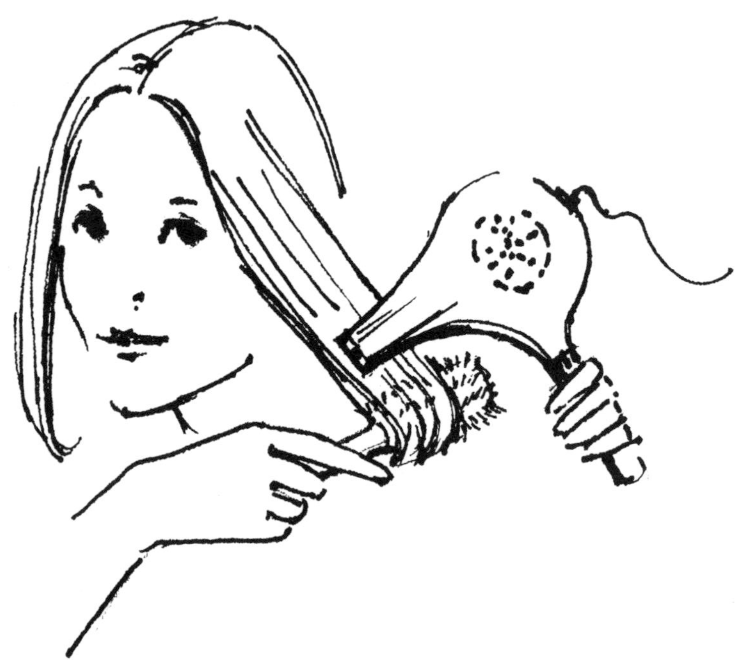

brush and hold it quite taut straight out from the head, as you dry it with the blower held in your other hand about six inches away. Keep the dryer moving steadily from scalp to ends as you brush.

If your hair is wavy or curly and if the final hair style you want has volume or bend or even curl and wave, then you should use a round brush. Dry the hair in sections just as if you were putting rollers in, holding it taut and turning it around the brush at the ends, holding it there a few seconds each time you brush.

If unblown hair dries out before you get to it, spray it with a little water or liquid setting lotion. You can keep the unworked-on sections out of your way and wet if you clip them up.

Never keep the dryer pointed at one spot too long or you'll scorch the hair. Keep it moving along with the brush.

Blowing the hair dry is easier to do on someone else, so you'll be in luck if you can enlist a friend's help. On yourself, you will have to get used to the strain of holding your arms up for quite a while and to wielding the brush, at least part of the time, with your left hand. You'll be able to manage after a few times. Hold the brush, not by the handle, but by the back, if it's easier for you.

Often, you'll want additional height or body somewhere on the

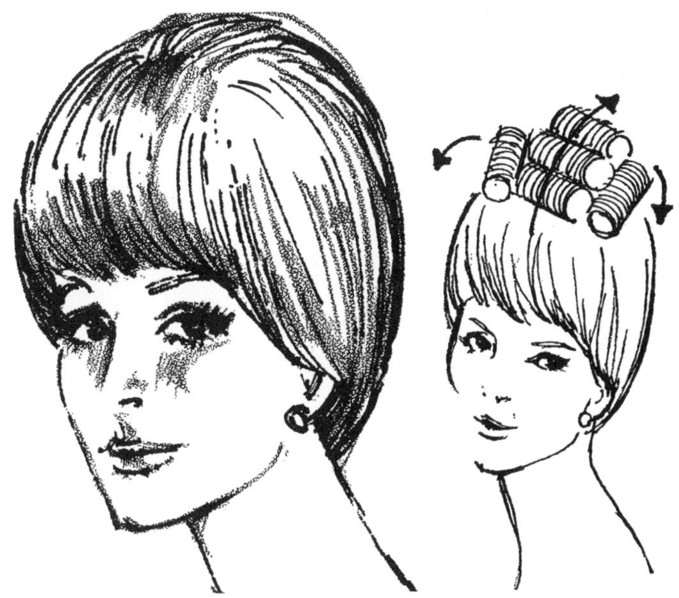

Short Summer Hair

head after a blow-dry setting. In that case, put that section up in electric rollers for a few minutes.

Occasionally a body permanent is helpful for hair that needs more substance or curl than you can get without a conventional setting.

Touch-Up Sets

There are quick sets to revive a hairdo that's lost its bounce. Never rewet your hair or you'll completely lose the line from your original setting. Set it dry. Follow the line of the setting with a few rollers or pin curls, and leave it for about an hour. Or, if you like,

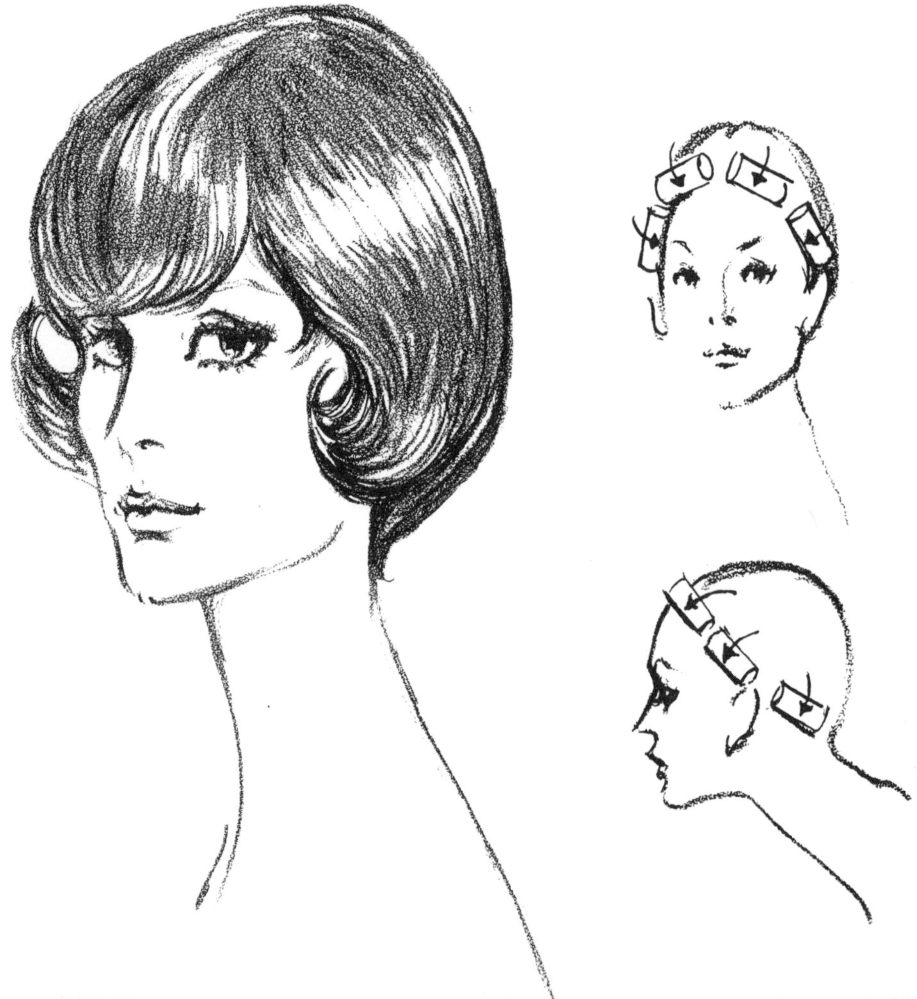

take a hot bath or shower and the steam will give it enough dampness so that when it dries your hair will have some body. Of course, you must know your own hair. Some people's hair is so porous that even the steam from the hot bath will make it so damp that they'll need to sit under a dryer for five minutes. Other people's hair will be dry by the time they put their makeup on.

If you need a bit more holding power spray a dry set lightly with hair spray, water or setting lotion and let it dry for about a half hour.

Another quick way: Dampen your fingers with cologne and run them lightly through the strand of hair you are rolling up.

You can use a hand blower to touch up a setting. Lightly spray the collapsed strands with hair spray. Dry the hair with the dryer as you comb the hair into big sausage curls, making them over and over until they are completely dry.

A curling iron will give shape to a curl that has loosened or straightened. I often use one in photographic studios when there is no time for a whole set or to wait for heated rollers to get hot. I'd suggest using the curling iron sparingly and carefully, as it will dry out the ends rapidly.

Of course, the heated rollers are designed specifically for quick sets. Read on.

Electric Rollers

The plug-in heated rollers are no fad—they're here to stay because they are extraordinarily useful. Mechanically, they work the same as ordinary rollers except that you allow them to heat up before using, and you fasten them in place with special hairpinlike holders. They were designed for pickup sets, to revive a drooping set, or to give yourself a little extra lift on the crown or curl at the ends. They were *not* designed for constant, every-single-day use. If you handle your hair this much, it can become dried out, split, unmanageable. About three times a week is fairly safe for normal hair and less for color-treated or dry hair.

Just remember that anything you do in excess can cause problems. If you take too many baths you get dry skin. If you drink too much you get drunk. If you heat your hair too much it will get damaged. So save the heated rollers for the times when you really need them. Choose either the dry or the steam rollers. And always use electric-roller conditioner or treatment-setting lotion with them to keep the hair from drying any more than necessary.

Most of the electric rollers are made with bumps to make the hair easier to roll. I've found that people tend to roll their hair sloppily, and when they take out the rollers the hair tangles and breaks. Unroll the hair carefully, straight down and slowly. If you like, you can file off the bumps a bit as many models have done.

Put the first rollers in at the crown and work down. When you unwind, take out the bottom rollers first and work up to keep hair from tangling too much. Always let the hair cool before you brush it to help "set" the set.

Electric rollers must be used differently on different kinds of hair. If yours is very fine and straight, you can give some body to it with the heat if you roll up smaller sections of hair per roller, dampen the hair just slightly before you roll, and leave the rollers in until they're completely cool.

Naturally wavy hair can get more lift and control from electric curlers if you use the largest rollers and remove them fairly quickly.

Color-treated hair is fragile and can't take too much handling. Neither can permanented or straightened hair. Always use the electric-roller conditioner, and remove the rollers *before* they're completely cool. Use the heated curlers *only* when absolutely necessary, never more than once a week, and use them only in the places where you *must* have curl or control.

Wrap Set

Wrapping your hair around your head is a good way to "set" hair straight and give it a good finish. It will help to keep it stretched out of its own curl or wave pattern. You can do it after a shampoo or

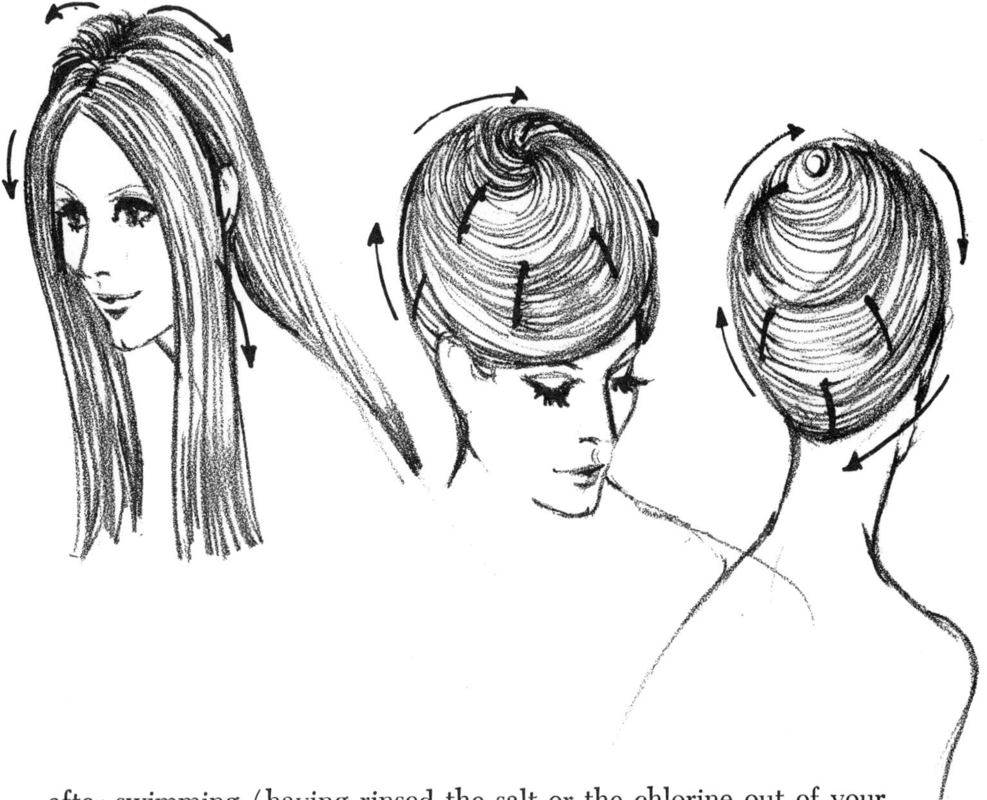

after swimming (having rinsed the salt or the chlorine out of your hair, of course) and let it dry in the air.

First, towel-dry your hair and comb it straight. Divide it into four sections by making two parts, one from the center front hairline to the nape, the other from ear to ear.

Take one section in the front, comb it across the part and into the second front section, wrapping it around the head like fabric, pinning it with bobby pins as you go. Remember that you must keep combing while you're wrapping to keep the hair very smooth.

Now take the second section and do the same thing in the same direction. Then do the same with the last two sections, combing each one into the other.

In other words, wrap the hair around your head like a flat turban, pinning as you go, with each section combed right into the next.

Special Sets

Some women—and hairdressers—have found individual ways of setting hair because of a particular problem, a particular hair style or a particular look they want to achieve. Settings can be washed right out so you can always experiment. A good idea may occur to you if you think of setting as a way of arranging your hair the way you want it to be when you comb it out.

Here are a few "different" ways to set your hair:

ALL PIN CURLS: This is especially good for women who are trying to grow out layered hair styles and have an interim period when their hair is neither here nor there.

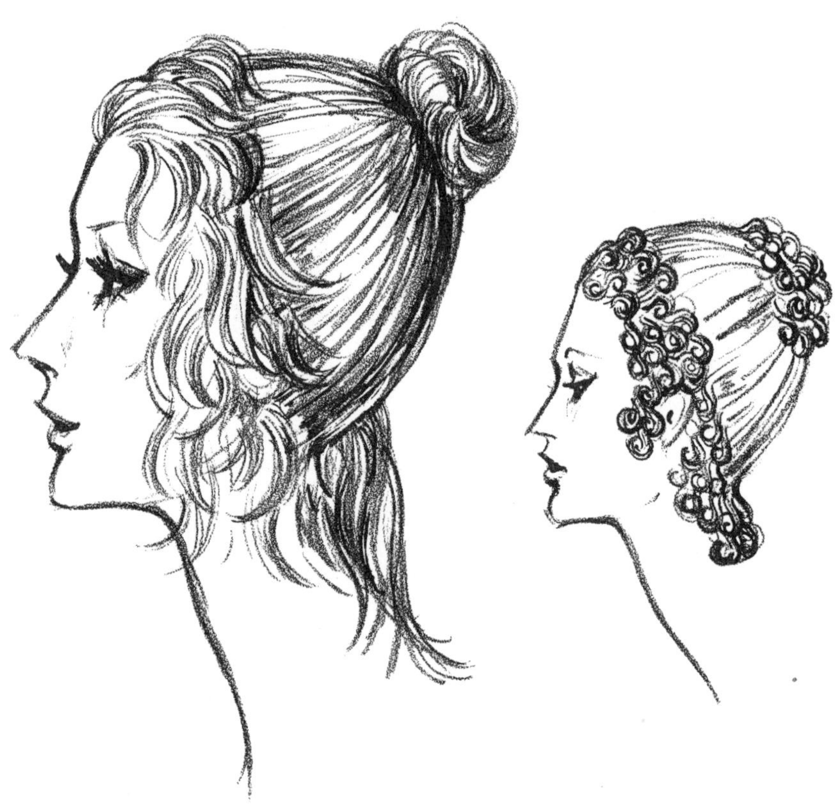

PERMANENT-WAVE RODS: To get very thick, kinky, curly hair—a look that's currently popular among young girls—you can set your hair on tiny permanent-wave rods. While the setting pattern is much the same as a roller setting, I always wind the front hairline rods toward the face because this produces a better finish around the face.

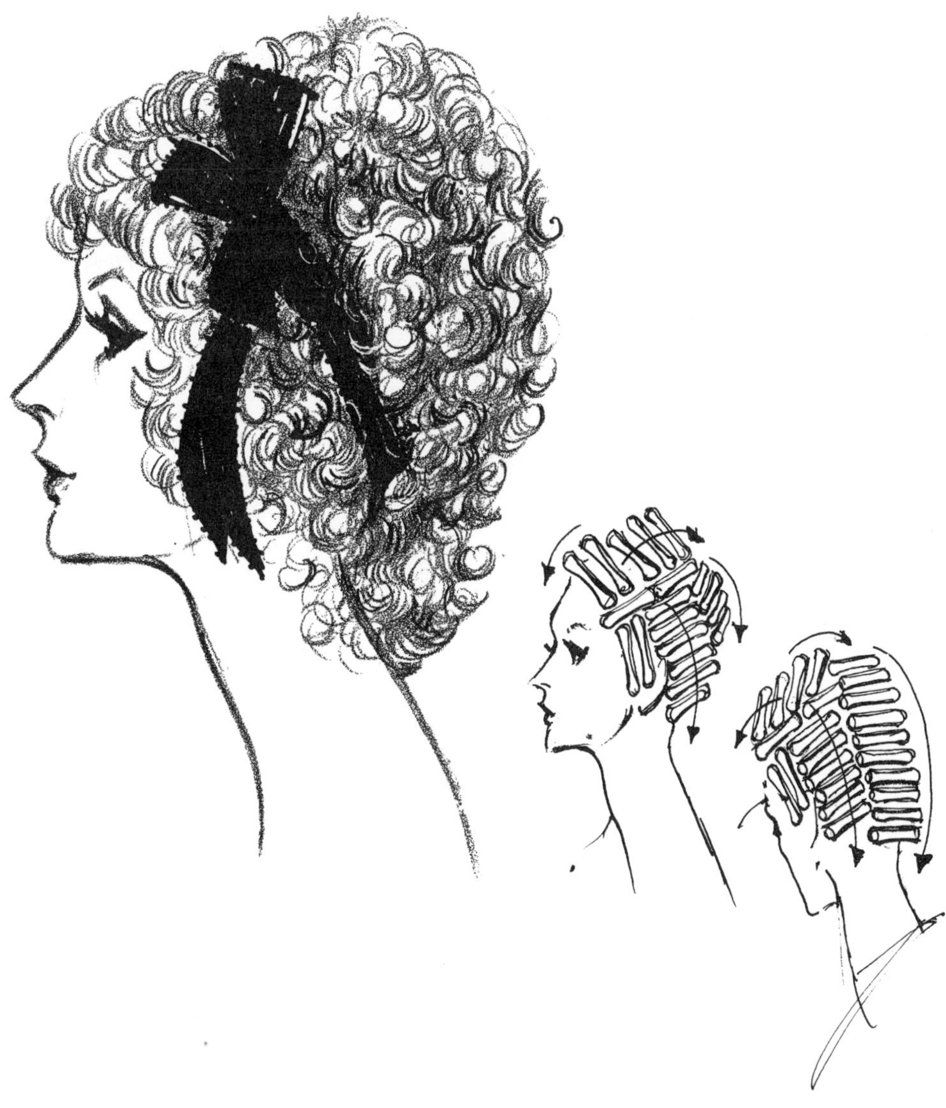

ENDS ONLY: A woman with a strong wave pattern at the hairline who wants curl only at the ends, or is trying to control a voluminous amount of hair and wants it closer to the head, can try a setting like this. Here only the ends are set while the crown is combed straight.

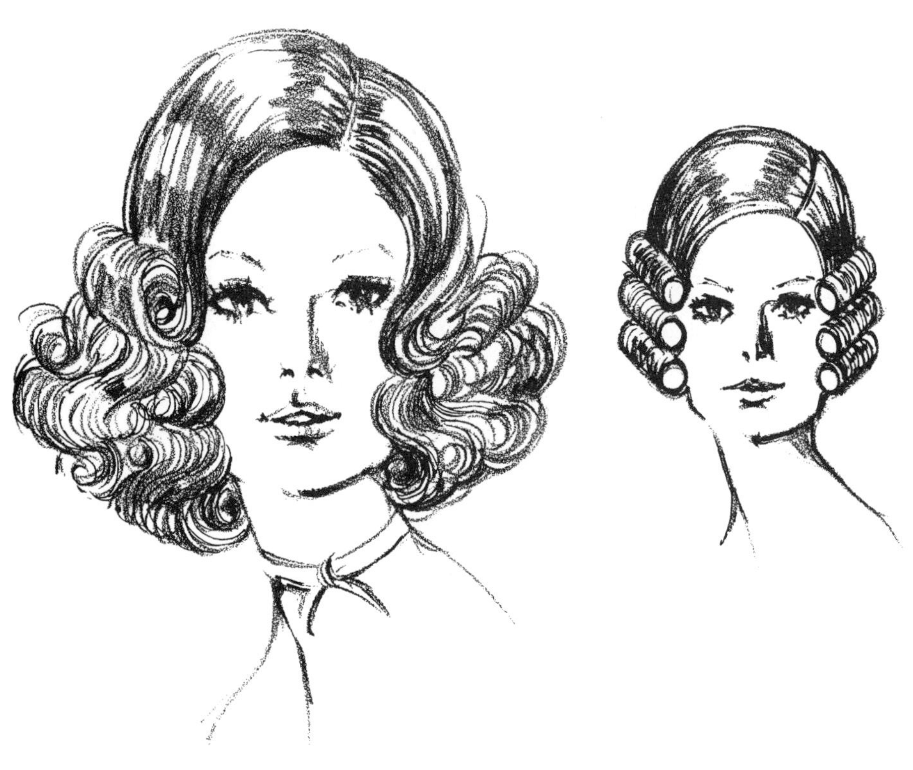

Chapter 6

CHOOSING A HAIR STYLE AND A HAIRDRESSER

New hair styles happen much less often than people think. What's often considered a new style is usually merely a variation of an old one, produced by setting or combing the hair a little differently. A truly new style comes only from a new kind of *cut,* a rare occurrence. Hair styles are never "created"—in spite of what hairdressers would like you to think—they *evolve.* They evolve right out of the recent past and will change into something else tomorrow, helped along by mechanical and technical developments.

To show you what I mean, let's explore recent hair history. Until the '50s, hair styles were not very pretty. Women wore hats for flattery and only had their hair washed and ironed and maybe curled on the ends. About 1955, the Italian cut came along, the first big change in years. This was three to five inches of layered hair all over the head. It was set on rollers about a half inch in diameter to give volume—a brand-new idea—and brushed out and worn rather curly. Every other woman wore this hair along with the waistless chemise dress.

They discovered with the Italian cut that the rollers gave their hair a lift which they found more flattering than the flat hair styles they'd been wearing. It was a break-through.

The Italian cut evolved into the Bubble, which was the same haircut set on larger rollers, perhaps three-quarter inch or even an inch or an inch and a half in diameter. The Bubble often had bangs

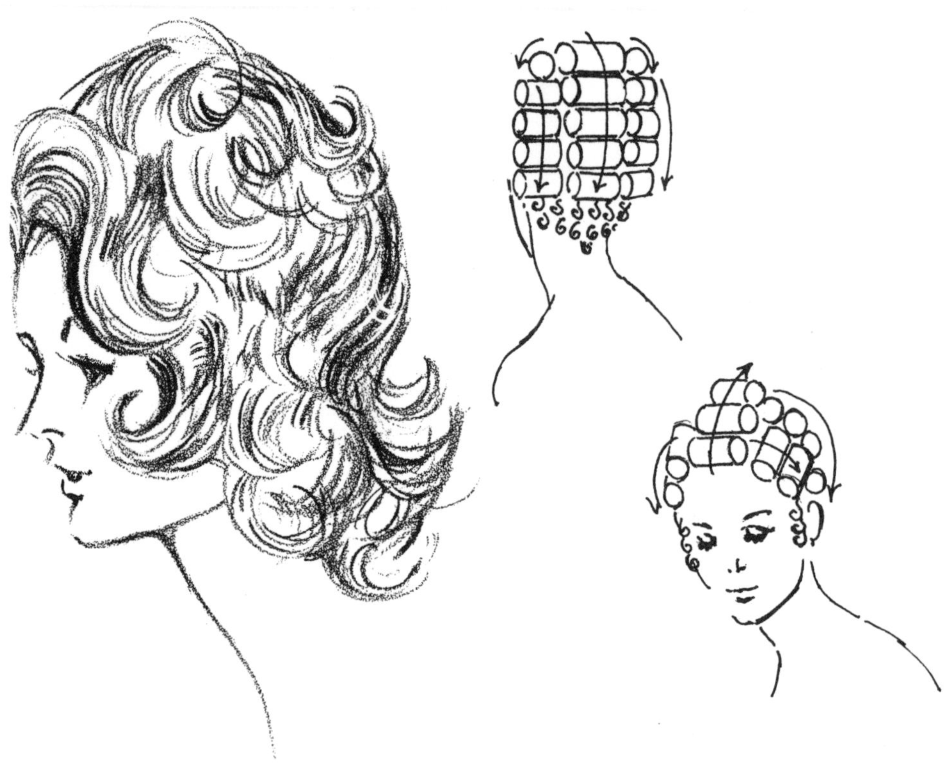

set on rollers to give them a smoother look. During the era of the Bubble, the first wigs appeared, shaped, of course, the same way.

Because women were not yet into cutting their hair on a regular schedule, their Bubble hairdos grew longer—and turned into the Bouffant. This was longer hair set on larger rollers. It was usually turned under because it was layered hair in various stages of growing out, though later, as the ends grew into more different lengths, they began to be flipped up to hold them together.

The Bouffant turned grotesque for a while as it grew bigger and bigger, helped along by the revival of teasing and spraying. Women would have their hair done in a huge mass produced by massive snarled and teased hair covered over with smoother hair on top and sprayed into cement. Then came the Beehive, which was a big teased Bouffant with a French twist.

Extra hair, either real human hair or synthetic, which started

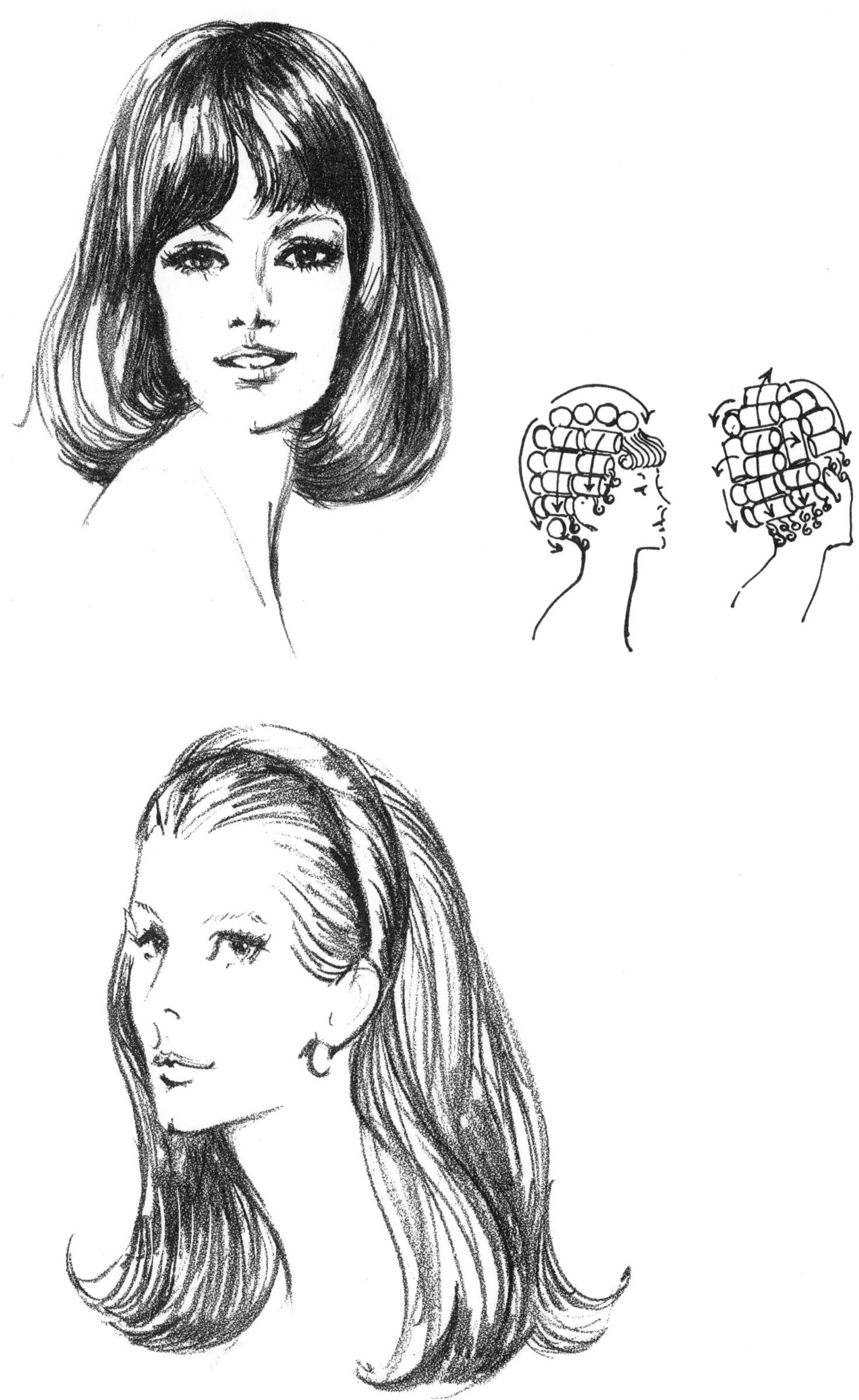

making tremendous progress toward looking real, became almost a necessity for people with poor hair who wanted the look of a lot of hair like everyone else. Soon even those with good hair wore the fakes. The fall came first. It was fairly short and was used to give volume. Then came the wiglet which was essentially a filler for the Bouffant.

An extension of this was a period of Louis XVI styles in terms of coiffures, hairdos that were very complicated and intricate, some requiring the daily attention of the hairdresser to keep the two or three or even four hairpieces in control, and the extras in place—braids, added curls, clips and other decorations.

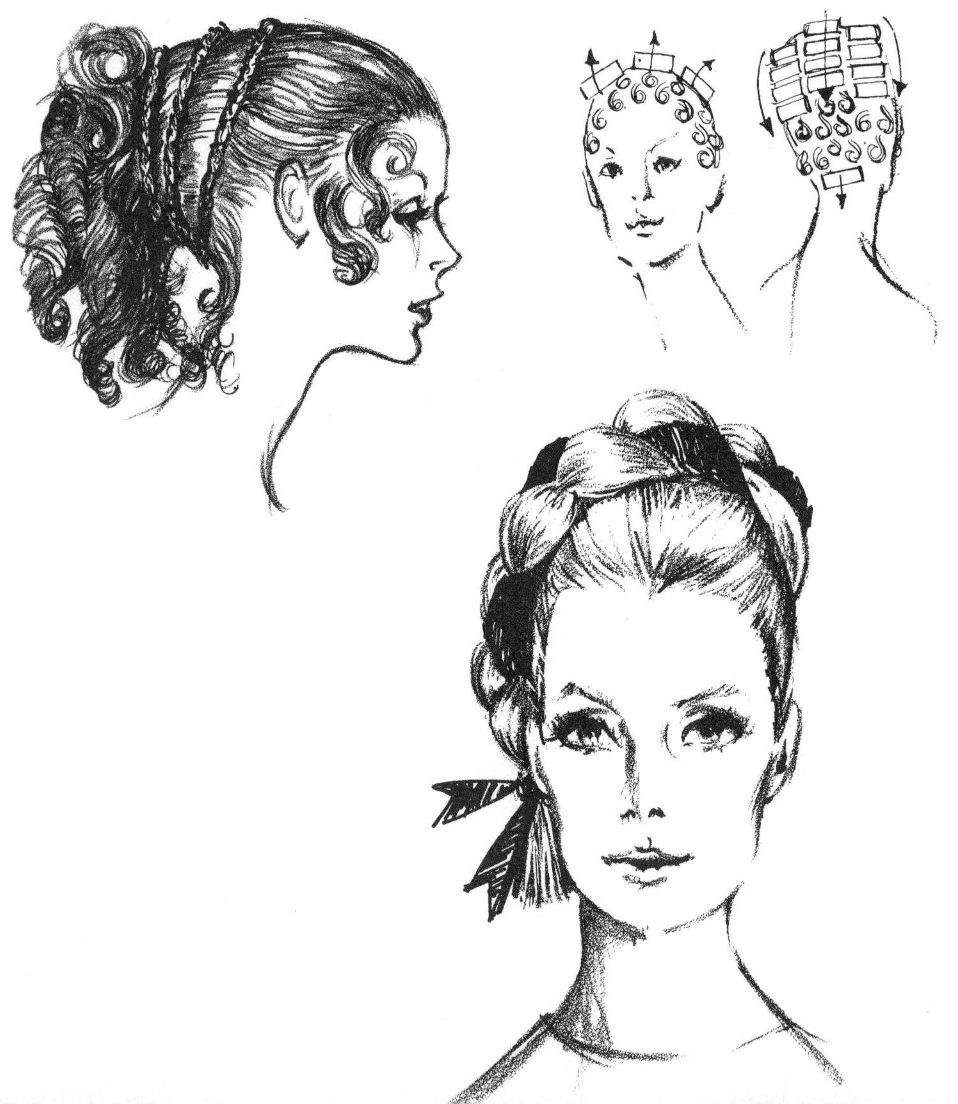

Hair had become *the* most important fashion accessory. Women liked the sense of a lot of hair. It made them feel feminine and luxurious and pretty.

Worn more simply, the grown-out hair of the Bouffant turned into chin-length hair cut in even lengths all around, though perhaps shorter in back and longer in front. It grew longer and longer and evolved into really long hair. As hair got longer and longer and longer, so did the fake falls.

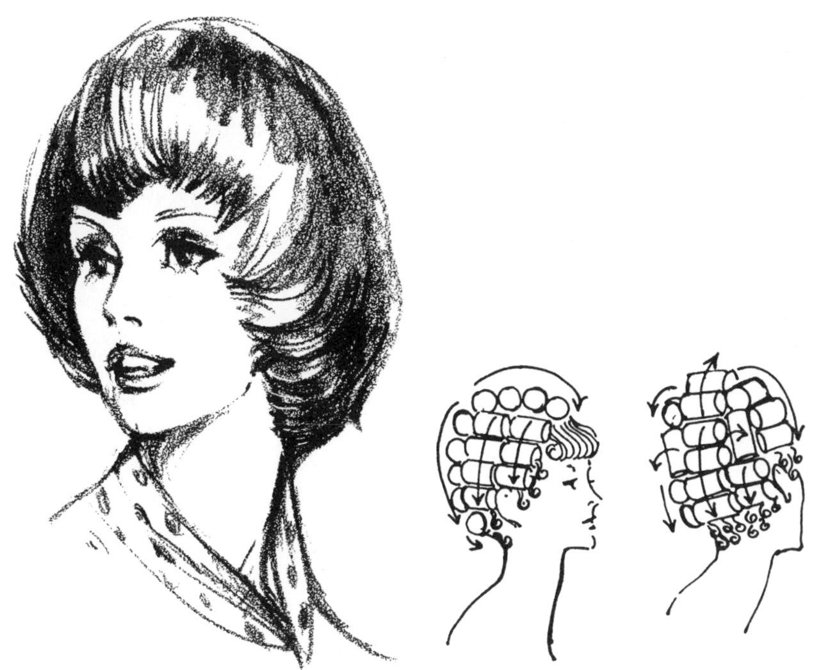

Women who weren't eighteen any more or who didn't like the way they looked with long hair wanted to do something more with it. Some tied it back into a George Washington style, which was teased for height or worn absolutely flat to the skull. Some cut shorter pieces of hair around the face for a two-layered effect.

Or they had it cut into a basic Serf shape—non-layered hair which went from short around the face to long in the back without any big jumps.

Some girls began to curl their long hair, sometimes with permanents, sometimes just for the day.

The curl led into a desire for shorter, curlier hair, and again we began to cut hair and developed the first big change since the Italian cut. This is the long-short or short-long hair, sometimes called the Napoleon or the Shag, which is layered hair that is much shorter in the front than in the back.

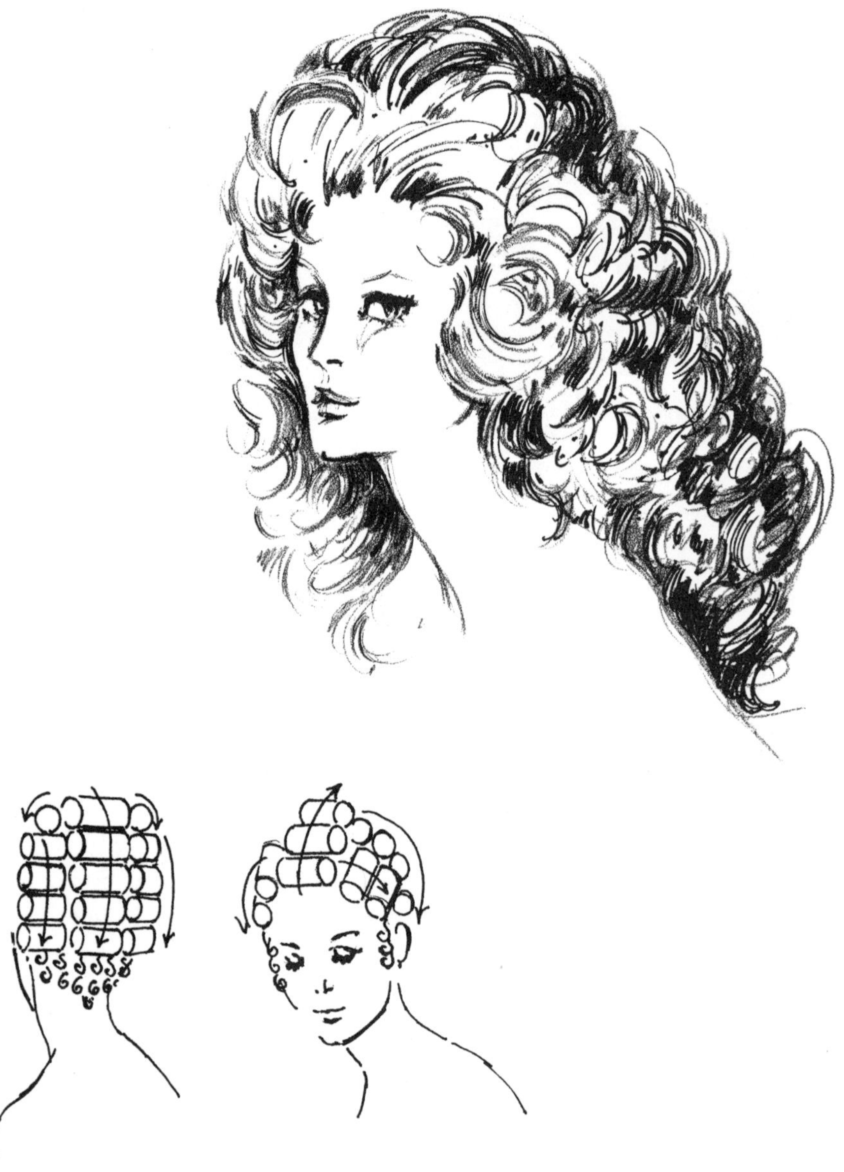

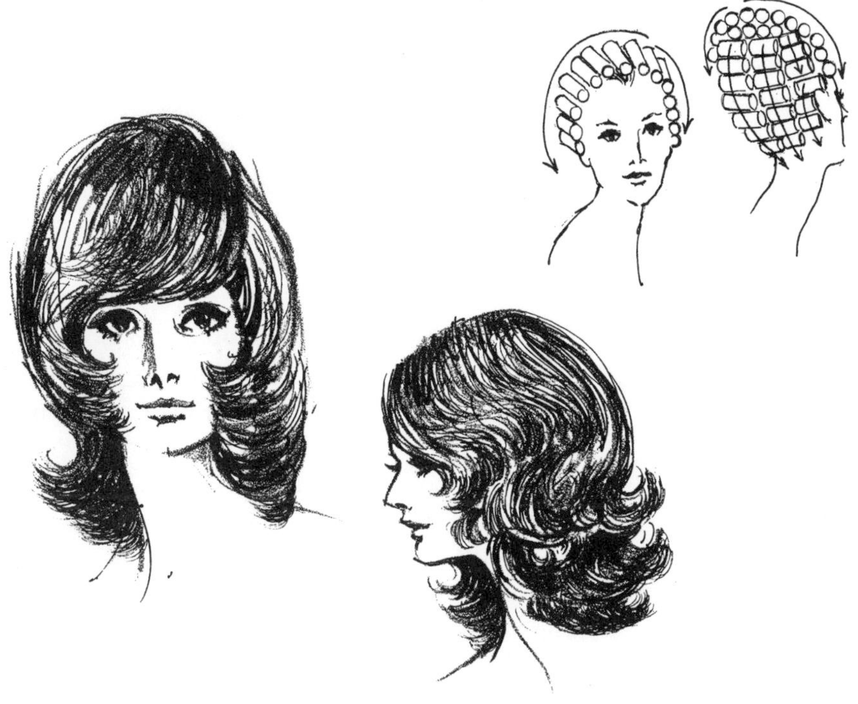

Now that is fading, and we are into much more all-one-length hair, usually blown dry and depending absolutely on the perfect haircut and good healthy hair.

Good haircuts as the basis of hair styling are going to lead, I think, to a future in hairdressing that isn't going to be too affected by people like me and my scissors. The future will depend mainly on break-throughs in science: the discovery of why we lose hair and how to prevent it; how to change the texture of the hair one has; how to keep the color and not go gray; how to get a different color without dye. All these are where the future of hair is.

Interestingly enough, through all of these modifications in the look of hair since the '50s, *mass* hair styles haven't really changed since the advent of the Italian cut. We've been living for fifteen years now with what I can only call the great American hairdo, an outdated Italian cut, and most women, especially the older ones, are still walking around with it. It's short, layered, razor-cut, thinned a little or a lot, bodiless, permanented if possible, tinted or bleached to colors even your taxi driver would know for sure. And it's puffed up, teased unmercifully, carefully arranged, then sprayed into concrete. It's been done by a pastry chef, not a hairdresser.

A woman spends the entire week between visits to the hairdresser trying to preserve this ungodly mess by wrapping toilet paper around it at night, then putting a net on it. She wouldn't think of combing through it, but just adjusts the surface every morning. And she wouldn't allow anyone to muss it up.

I don't like it. In fact, I loathe it. There's nothing pretty or sensuous about this hair that's still worn by an awful lot of women today.

I don't think anyone should look as if she's just come out of the beauty salon. That's a terribly unattractive look. Hair should be hair, it should have the quality of looking alive. Truly beautiful hair is something you want to touch, not recoil from in horror, as I often do. To understand what I'm trying to say, walk down the street and see just which heads you would want to touch. I'd be willing to bet you'd choose the ones that look clean and healthy and free and natural.

The set that lasts a week and looks it is definitely *over.* A set should provide line and body. Period. I don't care if the set collapses immediately. People try desperately to get hair to look the same every day. I don't think it should look the same tomorrow as it does today. It is not a plastic thing that should be cast in a plastic form.

The reason, I think, that so many women across the country are still wearing their hair the way they did fifteen years ago—granted, with slight variations—is that we all tend to see ourselves within a certain framework. We are used to looking a certain way. How we look is a reflection of our conditioning, the way we grew up, the way our neighbors and friends look, what our family likes, the "life style" of the area in which we live.

Consequently, when a woman sits in a salon chair and we give her a part on the other side of her head, or we flip it up instead of under, she thinks there's been a major change. It's not a major change at all. It's a small one, but it makes a big difference, especially if she's been living for years with her hair worn one way.

You must try to get past your conditioning and your old habits if you want a hair style that is beautiful *today.* Try not to limit yourself to the patterns of your times and your town. Even hair with problems can be beautiful in itself—though it may not be possible within your idea of what is fashionable. It's not necessary, I feel, to look like everyone else on your block.

The great new hair fashion of today is *health.* This is a time of beautiful hair, luxurious hair, shiny hair, healthy hair. It can be long to the waist or an inch all over the head. It can be curly. It can be bone straight. What it must be more than anything else is manageable by its owner. That is where it's at today.

To my mind, a good hair style is one that looks good when it's wet, when it hasn't even been set. This is the direct result of an absolutely marvelous haircut that gives the hair a line, a shape, a memory. Then, no matter what you do to it or don't do to it, it's *something.* To me, that is what hairdressing is today. You wash your hair and you let it dry in a shape. You wash it and put three rollers on top for volume. You wash it and then blow-dry it and stick five or ten hot rollers in to curl it a little. You wash it and roll up the entire head on big rollers to smooth it out, or small rollers because you want to curl it, or pin curls because you don't want to go around in rollers while it's drying.

It has a shape.

It has a superb haircut. You don't have a chance for beautiful hair without one. So concentrate on getting it.

How do you get this superb cut? You need the best hairdresser in town, so spare no expense. The reason a hairdresser may be expensive is that he's selling time as well as talent. There are those who do forty cuts and sets a day. I say you can't do that many and do them well. In my salon, we take twenty minutes to cut and twenty minutes to set, and we lose more customers on account of the time it takes than on account of the way the hair is done or the expense. It takes time to go to a good hairdresser. You can't rush it.

People always ask what my favorite hair style is. I don't really have one—it's different for every single woman. And I really don't care about style, except that the hair should be clean and untortured. Whether it's straight or curly, long or short, simple or more "done" is up to you and your special kind of hair. Almost every woman can wear almost any hairdo within the realm of reason if it's proportioned to her head and body. Too many women think there's only one style for them. That's not true—I could show you infinite ways a woman could look great.

Your hairdo should do something for you, make you feel pretty. It should flatter you, make the most of your hair texture, curl and thickness. It should suit your way of life and be comfortable. It should look like it's part of you and not a piece of abstract sculpture sitting on the top of your head. And yet it should have a shape.

That's a big order, you say, and easy for me to recommend. But how do you achieve that kind of hairdo? How do you choose one?

Well, you can't pick one off the head of your best friend or off the pages of a magazine—though you can certainly use these ideas as an aid. Nor can you choose a style merely by the shape of your face—that's a hoax perpetrated by the "experts" and I think it is ridiculous. I suppose all faces have shapes, but I have always managed to ignore that fact—unless, of course, they are truly extreme. I have never fallen into the trap of hairdos for "face shapes" and I refuse to fall into it now. I've gone nearly twenty-five years ignoring all those "rules" because I think they were made for really very few cases and applied to many. Women are always being asked: Do you have a round face, a long face, a square face, a diamond-shaped face, a heart-shaped face, maybe even a pear-shaped face! Out of the thousands of women who have sat in my salon chair, I have rarely seen one that made me think: "Oh, there's a square face."

Just to get this subject out of the way, let's take those very few exaggerated cases with extreme face shapes and see if there are any separate answers. To me, there are not. If I see a gross exaggeration of a face shape my reaction is to camouflage it, hide it, cover it. No matter what it is. If you have a tiny receding chin get as much hair around your face as possible. If you have a big square face cut

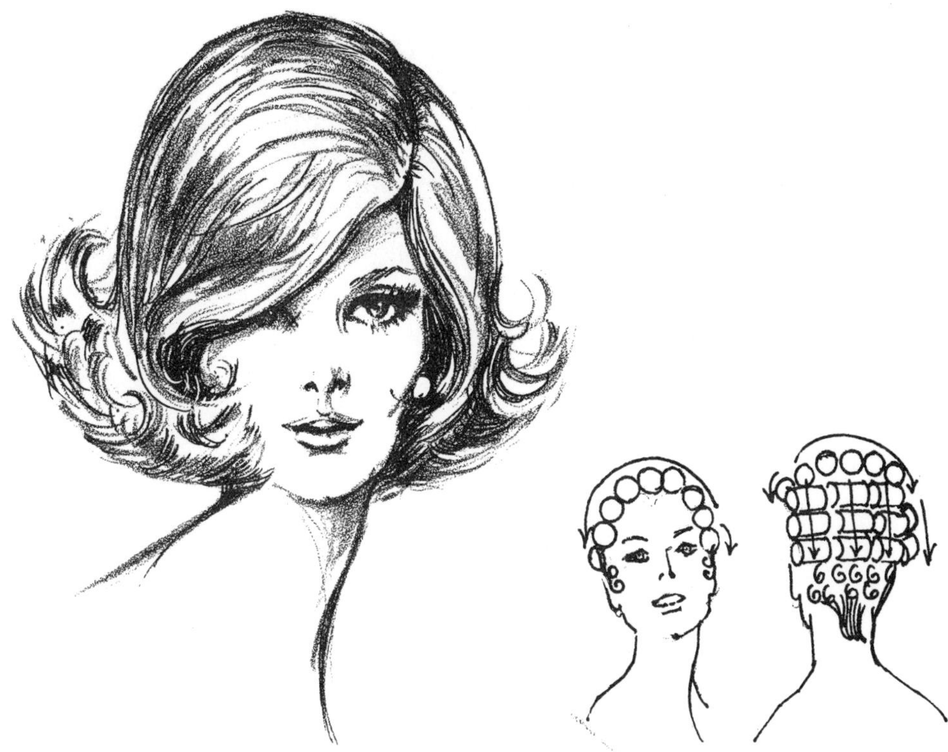

into it with your hair, cut it down. Bring your hair onto your face. If you have a long skinny face do the same thing.

Suppose you have a low forehead. If you uncover it you show everyone you have a low forehead. Wear bangs cut from way back and nobody will know what you've got under them. Of course, you could actually raise the hairline, if it grows very close to your eyebrows, by cutting or waxing away the unwanted area, or by the more permanent method of electrolysis. If you don't want to do that, start your bangs quite a bit farther back than your real hairline, so it looks as if your hair starts there.

The same answer applies to very high foreheads. Most women who complain about their high foreheads really have beautiful ones. But for those whose hairlines actually start beyond where the head starts to curve back, this *can* be a problem. If your hair is thick

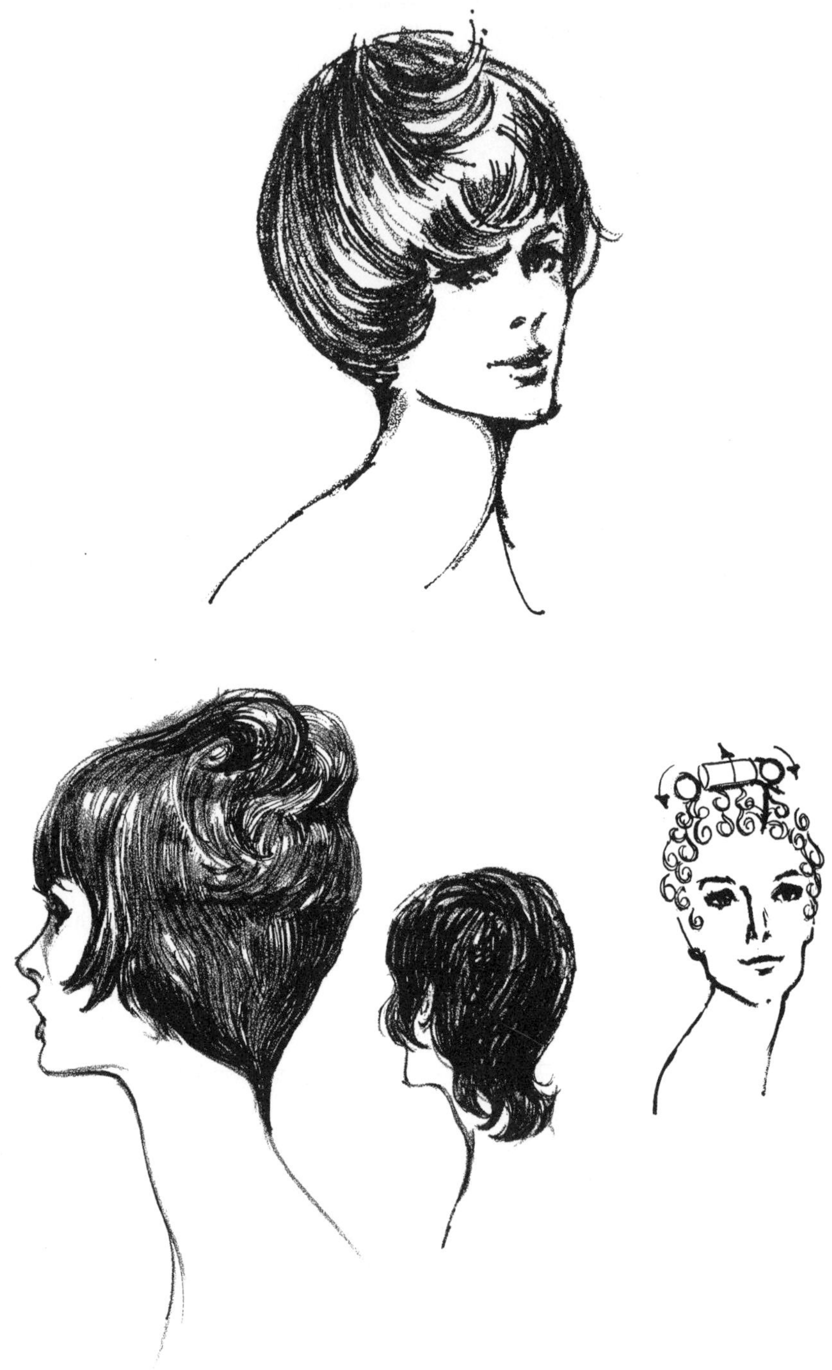

enough wear bangs as camouflage, again starting farther back than the hairline. If your hair is thin or fine, draped hair or hair that falls softly across the forehead to the side is a pretty solution.

Sometimes the hairline in *back* isn't the most attractive—either it's too high or too low. Suppose it's too high. If you have long hair, you don't have to think about it. If you want to wear short hair, though, you must always leave enough hair in back to give the illusion that it grows lower. For a very *low* back hairline, one that grows very far down on the neck, the solution is the same if you don't want to remove the excess hair.

I can tell you with honesty that almost everybody thinks her forehead is too high or too low. Almost everybody hates her nose. Almost everybody thinks her face is too fat or too thin, or too square or whatever. *I* don't think so very often, but *she* thinks so. Because she thinks so, she is led down the garden path of having to control her problems with a hairdo. In just about every case, it is nonsense. Except for those gross exaggerations, a girl with a round face or a long face can wear her hair pulled away from it and look great—*if* she is not hung up about it, *if* she has a kind of basic confidence.

Barbra Streisand is a good example of exactly what I'm talking about. She's worn myriad hairdos in the last five years. By the world's idiotic standards, she should try to camouflage her nose. But she looks marvelous—it's her attitude (and her makeup) that does the job.

More important than the shape of your particular face is the whole look of you. You are a combination of many things, not only a face shape, but a head size, a neck length, body proportions, height, weight, posture. Let's take somebody who has a long thin face. She may be 5 feet 2 inches with a long neck. She may be 6 feet 1 inch with a short neck. She may be very thin. She may be very fat. There are endless variations, all of which are elements in the way she looks and in the way she can do her hair.

How tall are you? Are you short-waisted or long-waisted? If you have a high, short waist, you're going to look disproportioned with very long hair. Is the size of your head in proportion with the width of your shoulders? The wider your shoulders, the smaller your head is going to look; the narrower your shoulders, the bigger your head will appear. Do you have a short neck? Then a solid mass of hair below chin level will emphasize that fact. Is your neck long? Then you'll probably look best in a longer style. How old are you? Unless you're eighteen or not much older, you can't wear your hair straight and hanging around your face. It needs a lift.

I've often seen a woman in a salon chair who looked marvelous in a big bouffant hairdo or a luxurious mane. Then she'd climb down and she'd be so short she could walk under furniture—a midget with a huge head. Or a woman with a tiny, tight, chic little head will stand up and turn out to be a giant who now looks like a praying mantis.

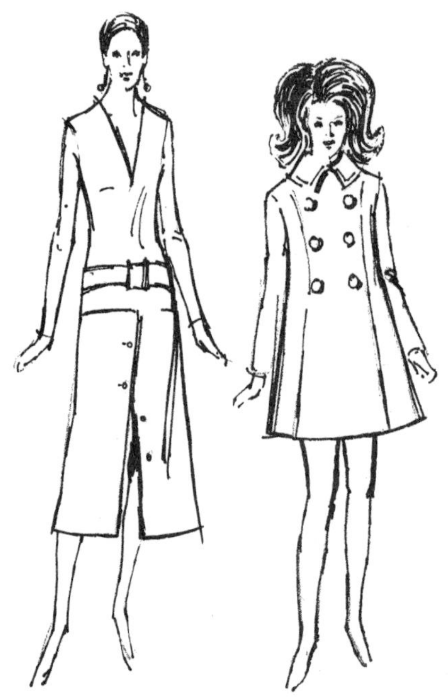

Each situation is entirely individual, however. I've seen tall thin women with very short tight hair who look great. Kay Kendall, for example, was tall and thin-faced, with large eyes and a long nose, a combination you'd never think would look good with a small hairdo. But her beauty was such that the exaggeration of a little curly, busy head was lovely.

And occasionally a little girl with big hair can be attractive. Nancy Sinatra, for instance, is a petite girl with very long hair. I like the way she looks because she has good proportions, plus a sense of security and spirit which allows her to carry it off.

Which only proves there are exceptions to every rule, even mine.

It's the texture of your hair that matters most in choosing a hair style. That's the material you have to work with, like the fabric of a dress.

You can't change the texture of your hair and so you've got to consider it carefully, work with what you've got. You must take what is yours and make it as good as possible—not into something else. Yes, you can make curly hair straight or straight hair curly, but it's temporary and may not be compatible with your hair. Understand your texture, the condition it's in, the curl that's in it or isn't in it, the good color or the unattractive color, the oiliness or the dryness. Be aware of yourself, *know* yourself. Is your hair fine or coarse or somewhere in between? Is it curly or straight or wavy? Is it thick or is it thin? Is it oily or dry or neither? If you don't work with what you have, if you don't choose a hair style which suits what you have, you'll become a slave to your hair and a slave to your hairdresser. And it won't be flattering anyway.

Hair texture, curl, its normal condition are inherited, along with hair color. As a general rule, lighter hair is finer in texture than darker hair. Usually, redheads have the coarsest hair, blondes the finest and brunettes are in between.

Let your hairdresser decide what problems your particular hair texture may present.

Hair without much body is better in a blunt cut than a tapered one. Hair which doesn't curl easily is best worn fairly short, or long and straight. If you haven't an abundance of hair you can't wear it long. If your hair is very fine and straight it should be cut in a style that will look good without any set at all. If it's very curly and you don't want to straighten it, it must be cut in a style which works with the curl, probably short and close to the head. If it's glossy and straight and coarse you can't have a curly style unless you want to work hard at it. Maybe you don't have any real hair-texture problem. In that case, you are very lucky because your hair handles easily.

There are other considerations too. I always ask, do you like your hair? How good are you with it? Can you set it, comb it yourself? How much time can you spend on it? Do you go to the hairdresser regularly? Are you a working woman? A housewife? A social type? Do you think it's important that your set lasts all week or do you prefer a softer look that may last only two or three days? What does your husband like or dislike? If you have a man chances are you want your hair to please him. (Of course, his hair should please you too.) Some men seem to have hang-ups about long hair, but most of them just want their women to be able to live without always crying, "My hair! My hair!" If you've got a hair style you can't relax with, it's got to go. It should require as little fuss and upkeep as possible.

I like to ask clients what they *don't* want, the kind of lives they *don't* lead, the kind of hair style they *can't* keep up with. I've discovered that I find out more about what they *do* want this way.

That's because most women know what they *don't* want and few know what they *do* want—that is crazy, but true. But if the hairdresser takes the time to find out a woman's taboos, they narrow down the possibilities and will often give a good and positive approach to the direction she should take with her hair.

I ask a client to tell me about herself. She tells me what is wrong with her—"I have a long nose. My hair won't hold a set. I have oily hair. My forehead is narrow." Very seldom does she tell me what's good about her. We talk about the texture and the curl of her hair. And her life style. "No, I haven't got a clue how to set my own hair." "I can't get to the hairdresser every week. I have seven kids." "I don't want a hairdo that needs a hairdresser every three days." Or, "I want that hairdo and I don't care how much effort it's going to take." We must both know what's best for her because a hair style that is out of context with her life style will only make her miserable.

Before you go to a hairdresser for a new hair style, you should know—at least, in general—the kind of look you want. Tell him what you want to look like. Take along a picture of a hairdo you like—that tells him what you think is pretty. Communicate your wishes to him and then be ready to listen to his advice. Together you will make the decision. You are partners in a hairdo. It is a matter of knowing yourself and letting the hairdresser in on the secret.

A hairdresser shouldn't be directed step by step, any more than a woman should ask, "How should I wear my hair?" and expect a specific answer. Each of you must contribute to a successful style. Discuss it. Most women, I've found, want to go into a beauty salon and have the stylist take over, giving them a magical solution to all their hair problems. Occasionally this works, but not often.

Don't go into a salon and say to the hairdresser, "Do what you think is best for me." That just won't work unless the two of you are intimate friends, because he might say, for example, "I think you'd look best with your hair pulled back off your face and tied in a knot on top. With the right makeup, you'd look terrific." Well, in the abstract, maybe you would look terrific, but perhaps you just don't see yourself that way. Maybe your husband likes pretty, fluffy hair around your face. Maybe you haven't the courage to have such a definitive hair style, or maybe you aren't the type to want to be made up properly all the time.

In other words, there is no *best* way for you—best is how it looks to you and how you can live with it.

Don't expect the perfect hairdo for you to happen in one visit to a new hairdresser. Plan on a second appointment at least and tell him what went right and what went wrong with his handiwork. Of course, you can't expect an exact replica of last week's hairdo. It never happens and I don't even try for it. I just try for the feeling of it.

If you don't like your hairdo when the stylist is finished with it tell him. He'd much rather you told him than all your friends. If he wants to keep you as a client he'll rework it.

Women think I am a magician. They think I'll say, "Oh, you must be a blonde" or "You have to have your hair cut off." I never say that, any more than I say, "How do you want your hair?"

I never talk anyone into cutting her hair, or straightening it or permanenting it, or coloring it. I may suggest it, but it's her head and *she* has to live with it. *I* don't. I tell her, "If you have *any* doubts about any of these irreversible steps, don't do it." A hairdresser must never force something on a client that she doesn't want. The name of the game is that she's happy and comes back.

People are always asking me how to select a good hairdresser. I always say, "Well, it seems to me the best way to judge a hairdresser is by his work. If you see someone on the street or at a party who has pretty hair or a good haircut, stop her and ask her who did it. Then, by all means, go to that hairdresser." Don't expect him to copy the hairdo exactly because your hair may be completely different. But explain to him that you like the feeling of Mrs. So-and-So's hair and you'd like to try yours in a similar way. Ask him if the style will work for you. And if he fails at first, don't give up on him; try again.

I have always found that hairdressers work best when there's a rapport between them and their clients. That's why I think every woman should have her own special stylist who, even if she sees him (or her) only a few times a year, will make her look pretty—which, after all, is the whole idea. If you've been running around trying one hairdresser after another I suggest you make a serious effort to find one you like.

I'm not saying you should stick with someone who doesn't please you. You should feel free to desert anyone who doesn't. Or if you find a salon you like but aren't satisfied with the particular hairdresser, don't be embarrassed about switching to someone else at the same place. Don't ever settle for routine work.

Unless you intend to go to the hairdresser at least once a week, don't select a style that is complicated. Intricate setting can't be done properly at home. Choose something simple and easy, something you can care for yourself. Gimmick hairdos need hairdressers. Caring for a simple hairdo is not hard.

Before you go to the hairdresser for a new style, do some homework. Play around with your hair and see what you think looks best on you. Brush all your hair back and see how it looks. Shake your head vigorously three times. Does it look pretty when it's free and tousled or do you need more organization? Brush it again, but to the side. Turn all the ends up. Then turn them under. If it looks too set, disarrange a few pieces of hair. If your hair is long, hold it so it looks shorter. Try it every way you can think of. Your eye will

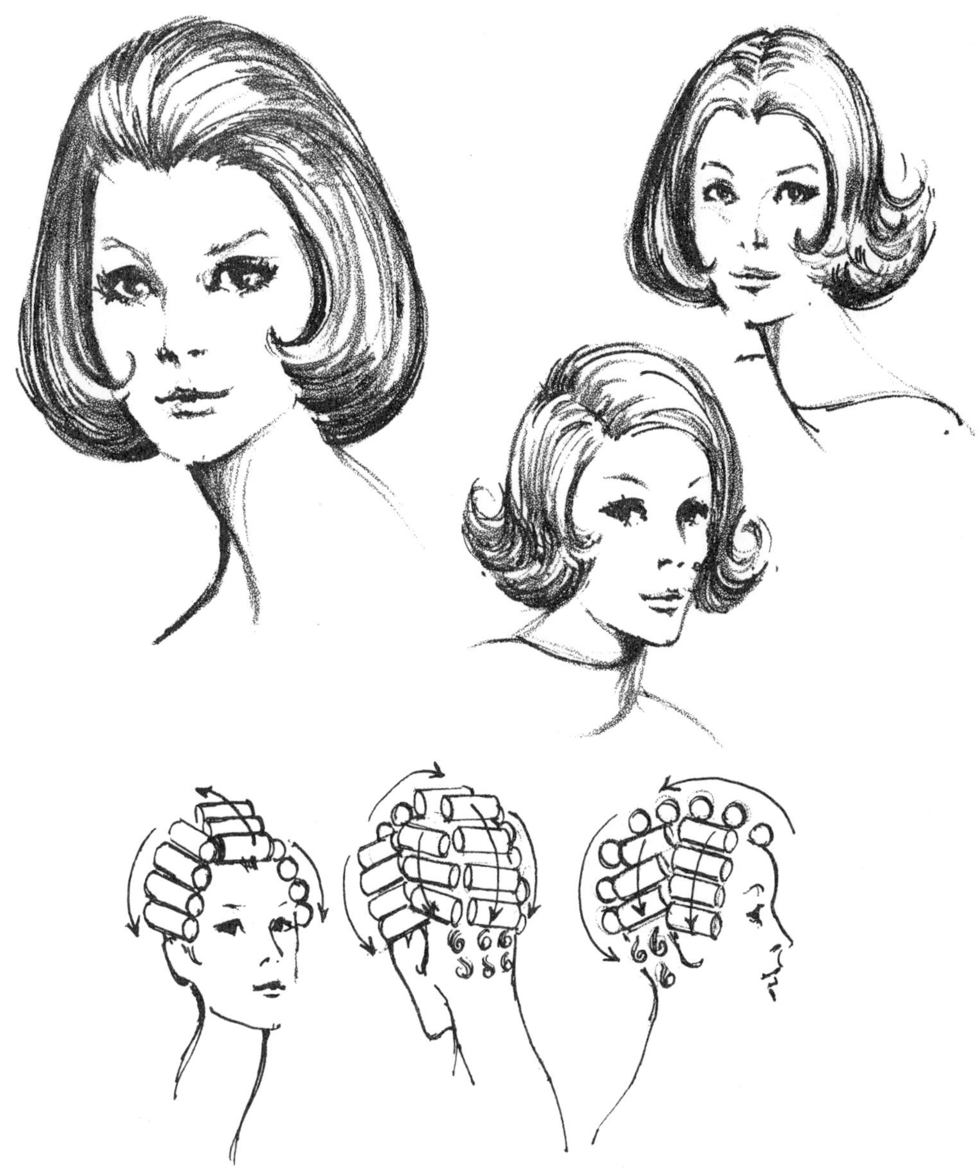

tell you when you've hit on a good effect—but remember to look in a full-length mirror for the total answer.

Another way to get a clue to hair styles for you is to try on some wigs in your hair color but in different styles. You might even buy one in the style you like best and wear it for a while before deciding what to do with your own hair.

Or the next time you shampoo your hair, fool around for a while with "shampoo sets." Work up a good lather of suds and then start experimenting, pushing your hair this way and that, giving yourself fake bangs or taking yours away, dipping hair over the forehead or brushing it back. Try parting it in different ways. See if you like yourself better with some height or fairly close to the head. This way, you may be able to get a good idea of a suitable hair style.

Often, when I go to a photographer's studio to do the models' hair for a magazine layout, I'm really doing the same thing. Each page has to look a little different, but the girl is the same. I've got five or ten minutes to change her hair between shots. I brush it from one side to the other, or straight back or down over the forehead, or up in front and down in back, and so on. There are myriad choices, and I keep changing until I hit on something I like.

Minor changes in hair are often major in effect. A part on the left instead of the right can make a big difference. Or perhaps combing the hair straight back rather than to the side can be spectacular. Try everything and see.

I suppose I do have to say something about tipping in a beauty salon. Frankly, I hate the whole idea of tipping—it's corruptive, both on the part of the person receiving the tips and the person giving them. And I feel it has kept a service from becoming a profession. I don't take tips myself, and I haven't for many years. I've lost a lot of money—maybe several thousand dollars a year—but I've had a satisfaction far beyond the loss of income.

I realize I'm not going to change the system, I can't fight it, and I can't tell you not to tip. When I first opened my own salon, I wanted to abolish tipping and add a service charge as they do in Europe, but the hairdressers were pretty glum about it and we realized that, no matter how we tried, we'd have women who would tip anyway, just as American women do in Europe. In fact, there are clients who try to insist on leaving tips for me even though I forbid it.

If you are going to tip I think you should base the amount on the service given, not just an automatic 15 per cent, which is the usual thing. If you are pleased with the service the tip should reflect it. If you are displeased the same is true.

P.S. I know. I haven't talked about hair styles for girls who wear glasses! There are no special hair styles for girls who wear glasses. I feel that you must not try to match your hairdo to your glasses. Pay no attention to your glasses. If you look pretty in a hair style *without* them, you'll look pretty *with* them. If you don't, then your glasses are wrong. Too many people have been buying glasses which they think of as "high style," but which are simply overwhelming. There is such a wonderful range of choices today that this is a shame. I would suggest buying a pair that is simple, unobtrusive, a pale color, and has the least amount of frame.

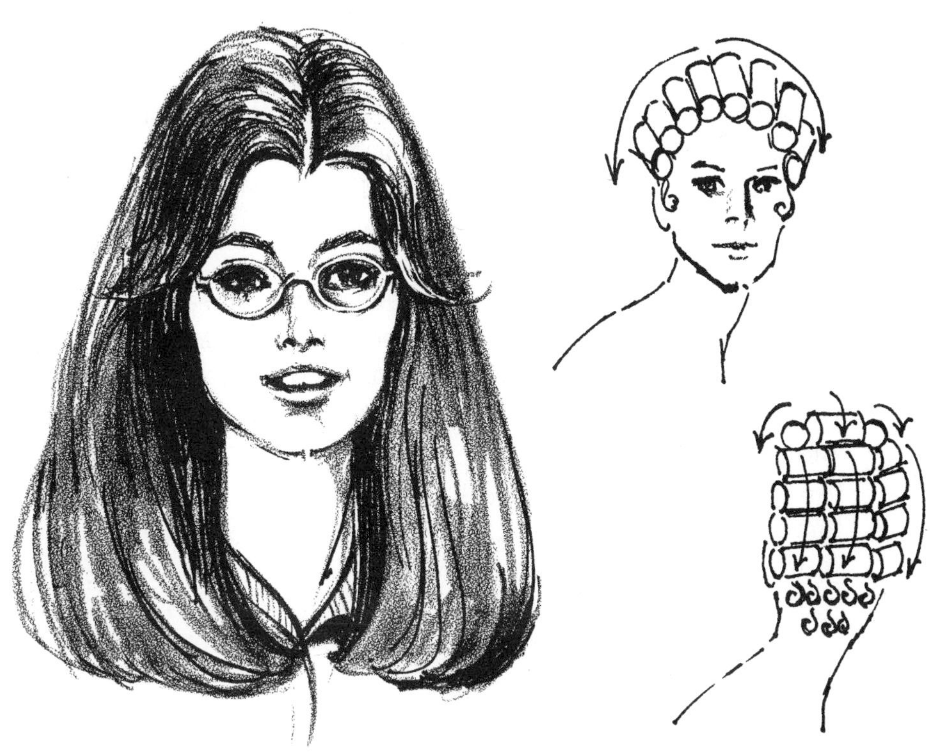

Chapter 7

HAIR COLORING

When I started in this profession almost twenty-five years ago, many women wouldn't admit even to their own families that they colored their hair. There were some "bleached blondes" and "bottle redheads" among the younger women, but most people who colored their hair were going gray and didn't want anyone to know it. Today women change the color of their hair the way they change lipsticks. It's been estimated that half the women over thirteen in this country do it, and only about half of these use coloring to cover up gray.

I think that natural hair—if it's a good shade—is more beautiful than any that could possibly be produced artificially. And it's generally healthier. It doesn't require all the special attention that tinted or bleached hair needs, and as it grows, it doesn't keep changing color.

But to have dull hair today is just dumb. If your natural-colored hair is not the prettiest shade for you, there is no reason not to change it—but, please, to a color that looks like it could have grown out of your very own head. I have seen some of the most incredible, unreal, phony colors on people's heads, colors that could never have been made by nature. For some unknown reason, despite the fact that there are such marvelous tints now available, some women seem to like—or at least accept—these hideous shades.

In the last twenty years, great strides have been made in hair coloring. Manufacturers have developed their products to the point where you can color your own hair at home and do a very nice job. (A very nice job the first time, at least.) Professional tints and bleaches, applied by an expert, can be perfection. Plain women have been changed into beauties with a change of hair color; and beauties have become great beauties. Done well, hair coloring can —as the ads tell you—turn you into a new woman.

But, and this is a big "but," it will change your life in other ways too. I'm not trying to frighten you out of changing your hair color, but I want to explain what it is you are doing to your hair. Once you have bleached or dyed your hair with a permanent coloring, it is yours. You are stuck with it. If you don't like it, you cannot go back again. You no longer have your natural hair and you never will until all the chemically colored parts have grown out—on an average of half an inch a month. You must retouch the roots every few weeks, you must take special precautions to protect your hair, and you must treat it gingerly. Bleach your hair and the natural pigment is forever gone from that hair that's been bleached. Dye it and the natural pigment is forever covered on the hair that has been colored.

Hair coloring has become so easy to do that we don't realize just how much we are actually doing chemically. It's amazing how few people really understand that. Advertising, which tells you that you can color your hair in five minutes and it's all so simple and don't you want to do it, makes you think you're not doing an awful lot. Something that easy, you feel, can't be much. But it *is*. And your life will now be different. That's why I suggest that you understand what you are really doing and why you are doing it.

When you change your hair color, you are bleaching and/or dyeing it. Bleaching is when you remove the natural color pigment of the hair. You decolorize it. Once this is done, it is permanent, whether you have removed a lot or a little of the pigment. When you go from very dark to very light hair, you must have your own color stripped away by bleaching, and then have some color put back in by tinting.

Tinting is when you add color to your hair by "coating" and/or penetrating it with dye. You cannot go lighter by tinting; you can only go darker. And keep in mind that "color on color makes color." In other words, you are adding color to hair that already has depth. If you choose a shade that matches your own, for example, you will not come out with your own color but one that is darker and denser.

The element of taste is terribly important in hair coloring and one that is almost impossible to describe in general terms. Every single person is different and really requires an individual consultation. You will look good in some colorings and awful in others. It all depends on your skin tone.

Now that I've said I can't be specific, I'll try to be anyway. If your skin tone is very white, it would probably be best to exaggerate your own natural color. A very pale complexion needs a warm, not too pallid, color. If your skin tone is yellowish, you will be most unattractive in brassy or reddish hair colors. Light, ashy, subdued shades will probably be good. If you have a ruddy complexion, you'll exaggerate it by making your hair too deep, too strong, too red. The tone-on-tone approach is probably better than all one color for you. An olive or dark skin looks best with a darker hair color, not too deep but in the brown range, with, perhaps, golden highlights.

Another consideration in choosing a color is your age. As you get older, your skin tone becomes paler. So, you'll look best in hair that is not too dark and too much of a contrast with your skin. Generally speaking, as you get older, make your hair lighter than its original natural shade.

Few women, no matter what their ages, look their best with a minor color change. If they go only a few steps up or down the color range, they end up looking all one color, skin and hair, which is not flattering. That is because very few people, at least in this country, have distinctive coloring. Not everyone is an Elizabeth Taylor with pale skin, dark hair and violet eyes. As a result, what happens too often is that by making only a slight color change you still have the same lack of contrast, giving a monotone effect which I don't think is terribly attractive. That's one reason streaking is so successful. It gives an exaggerated color change and yet has some relationship to one's own coloring.

Probably the best way to find out how you'll look is to try on wigs in the colors you think you'd like. Don't even think about the style; you have to get past that. Just think about the color. Even better would be to buy a wig in your chosen color and wear it for a while.

Never make a drastic change until you're absolutely sure what you want. Change your color gradually, or stay close to your own natural shade. If you're over forty, don't try for the color of your hair when you were twenty. Now you must go into lighter, softer tones—anything too dark or too red is hard-looking and aging.

With a new hair color, you may have to examine your makeup, as there will be new reflections on your skin. Perhaps you'll need a brighter lipstick or a paler one, a different eye shadow. We turned a blonde into a redhead just the other day. She had very pale skin and had always worn blue lid color. With the red hair, the blue suddenly looked too strong and harsh, and I suggested she try a mauve or violet shade for a softer effect.

On the other hand, I don't want you to think that you can cure an unflattering hair color with makeup, especially today when makeup is no longer a mask. Your skin tone will remain just what it is; your hair color must look good *before* you put on the makeup, which will merely enhance it. If it doesn't you've chosen the wrong shade of hair. Just think of all the sallow-skinned girls you've seen in brassy blond hair. No makeup in the world is going to keep them from looking green.

Your own hair color is never solidly one shade. There are always variations from strand to strand. With the techniques and materials available to the colorist today, you don't have to have solid hair. It's always prettier and more real-looking to have a few shades, and especially to have the hairline a little lighter than the rest. The ultimate look today is what I call tone-on-tone. It may be five different but closely related shades, all ending up looking superbly natural. The tone-on-tone look, though, is nothing you can try at home. It requires a professional's expertise.

Streaking or shading is the way to color your hair without going all the way. This way, you color or lighten certain strands of hair all over your head, or just around the face. Shading gives a lift to your hair color without basically changing it. You look as if you've been out in the sun. It looks real and it's pretty, and it doesn't have to be touched up every few weeks as an allover color does. The real virtue of streaking is that there is no sudden change. Most women do themselves a disservice by going from one hair color to another that's totally different, sometimes destroying their own individual quality. I remember one movie in which Lana Turner was suddenly a brunette. I had always liked her wonderful blond looks and, to me, she just didn't look like Lana Turner any more, even though I knew her natural color was darker.

Shading must be done by a professional colorist in order to get that sun-streaked look, unless you are particularly skilled yourself.

If you make a mistake in hair color, what can you do? That's different for everyone. But, in general, if you've lightened your hair by bleaching it, you can now tint it darker. If it's been colored, the color can be removed by a process called "stripping" which is bleaching off the new color. This will not only remove the color you have added but your own as well, and you must have a new coloring job. The danger is that this will lead you down the garden path of constantly-taken-care-of tinted or bleached hair.

If you get to the point where your hair is really in terrible shape from pouring one thing after another on it, get yourself to an expert colorist to bail you out. Stop fooling with it yourself or switch from your inept colorist to a really good one. Sometimes I've had to tell people whose hair had become so damaged by excessive bleaching and coloring that they must just leave it alone, and let it grow out because any more chemicals might do away with it altogether. Grow it out, wear a wig in the meantime, cut it in a short style when there's enough length to your own virgin hair, and be more careful in the future.

When you go to a professional colorist, your responsibility ends after you've chosen him (or her). You are in his hands, so make sure he knows what he's doing before you give yourself to him. If you want to do your own coloring—and many women today do—then I ask that you learn how, first, to read labels. Some products are perfection for virgin hair, but are not meant for chemically treated hair (permanented, colored, bleached, straightened). Others are for certain shades or textures and not for others. READ THE LABELS.

Next, follow the directions to the letter. Manufacturers have spent thousands and thousands of dollars on research and development and have perfected their products so that they will work beautifully if you do *exactly* as they tell you. Each product is different, each is applied differently. READ THE DIRECTIONS. If you don't understand something or you are not certain that you have chosen the right product, don't use it. Write to the manufacturer—or call if you live close to the source—and you will find that the company will be happy to give you advice. If you have a problem after using a product ask the firm for advice and help. Many manufacturers operate hairdressing institutes and if you live near any of them, you can go there to have your hair-coloring problems remedied.

Do-it-yourselfers should stick to simple hair-coloring formulas, the one-process colorings, and temporary rinses. More complicated operations are best left to the professionals.

Don't do any experimenting on your own. I can assure you that you'll be sorry if you do. I've seen some of the results of experimenting. So have you, I'm sure. All products are not necessarily compatible. You usually can't, for example, mix two shades from two different manufacturers. And sometimes you can't mix two different shades from the *same* manufacturer. Perhaps they combine chemically, but like mixing oil paints or watercolors, if you don't understand color mixing you'll end up with muddy tones. Or you'll find yourself getting green highlights or too much blue or whatever.

Remember that some of the worst hair problems can be caused by misuse of coloring. Used properly and carefully, coloring is a boon for women whose hair is mousy, or fading or prematurely gray or just not pretty. Used carelessly, you're in trouble.

P.S. Hair coloring or bleaching can often, as a fringe benefit, have a good effect on the condition of your hair. If your hair tends to be baby-fine and limp, coloring can give it more body, help it hold a set better. If it is oily, it may well become drier and more manageable, at least for a while. If your hair naturally tends to be dry, condition it before and after you color it.

Now I will get off the soapbox and talk about the kinds of hair colorings there are. Basically, they fall in three groups: temporary, semi-permanent and permanent. The products usually will be clearly marked so that you will know whether you are getting a temporary or a permanent coloring agent. In general, temporary rinses are to be poured on and are marked "temporary." The label on semi-permanent rinses will specify the number of weeks or shampoos the color should last. On the permanent coloring packages, you will note that it says "shampoo-in hair color," or "creme formula," or the directions will call for the use of a "developer" which is generally peroxide.

Temporary Colorings

These are rinses which add color by coating the surface of the hair shaft like paint. They are applied after the shampoo. Some are poured on, some are sprayed on and some are even stroked on with a pad. This coating washes off with the next shampoo. You cannot lighten your hair with a temporary rinse; you can only darken it or change the tone, perhaps adding highlights. You are not changing the basic natural hair color. Pour some ash-blond rinse on brown hair and it won't work. But you can pour black rinse on brown hair and it will.

Even with temporary rinses, you must understand that the old rule, color on color makes color, operates here too. If you put a brown rinse on brown hair you will get a deeper brown. So, if you want to produce your own color to cover some gray, perhaps, choose a shade just a little lighter.

Do not expect 100 per cent coverage with a temporary rinse,

especially the first time you use it. If you use it on a regular schedule you will probably get some build-up and maybe almost 100 per cent coverage.

The nice thing about a temporary rinse is that if you don't like it you can just wash it out. You can brighten up your hair without a drastic change. And it's fantastically easy.

On the other hand, cautious Kenneth must warn you that, ideally, you will be using the rinse on virgin hair, hair that's been untouched by any chemical process. If your hair has become porous from permanent waving, or straightening or another kind of coloring, it can very well absorb even a temporary color and you may not be able to get it out.

Last caution: Even temporary rinses can affect the way a permanent wave will take. Stay away from the rinses at least two weeks before and after a permanent.

A handy use for a temporary rinse is as a toner. If you've bleached or streaked your hair without a toner you'll find that oxidation will often produce unattractive gold or red highlights. A temporary rinse in an ashy tone can help to overcome this color. (Problem: Most ash tones are based on blue. If your hair is *very* yellow it may turn green!)

Semi-Permanent Colorings

These are rinses which coat the hair and also have some percentage of penetration of the hair shaft. The effects last about four or five weeks and gradually fade away. These give more coverage than temporary rinses, especially for gray hair, and are applied after the shampoo, left on anywhere from a few minutes to a half hour, then rinsed out.

Semi-permanent products, too, will only darken or highlight the hair, never lighten it because they contain no bleach. They can add rich highlights or take them away; they can provide a rich color in place of a mousy one; give a golden glow to dirty blond hair; cover up gray hair—all within your own natural shade range. But they will not make your hair lighter.

Most have a cream-base formula which has a tendency, for the first week or so, to make the hair very, very soft—a problem for many people. After a rinse, if you have very fine or limp hair, a setting will probably drop right out within a block of the door on a damp day.

And the color will be just a little different every week as it gradually disappears.

Again, if your hair has been made porous by other chemicals it may absorb even this color permanently.

Both temporary and semi-permanent colorings are for women who don't want too much change, don't want to go through constant touch-ups, don't want to become slaves to hair coloring. They are quick, easy and not that much of a commitment.

To get rid of a semi-permanent color that you don't like, you can wait for three or four or five weeks until it fades away. Or you can speed up the fading process by a lot of shampooing in quick succession. Also, most of the manufacturers of semi-permanent rinses make removers to help take the color off. Henna is having a revival. This is a vegetable product that coats the hair shaft. It often adds red highlights, body and quite a nice sheen to the hair.

Permanent Colorings

Permanent colorings penetrate the hair shaft and cannot be removed except by cutting off the hair. You can change the color of your hair forevermore with permanent colorings, make it much lighter or much darker, cover the gray completely, make dramatic changes or simply heighten the natural color. As your hair grows, the new hair must be touched up every four weeks or so to match the already-treated parts.

ONE-STEP PERMANENT COLORING: This—the only kind to use at home—is available in two types. One is the "shampoo tint" which is bleach and color combined in one product. It is applied like a shampoo and both lightens and tints the hair at the same time in a single procedure. With a shampoo tint, you can start off with dark hair and go to lighter hair, maybe up to three shades lighter.

The second kind of one-step permanent coloring is "tint," once referred to as "dye." Tints are not shampoo-in colorings and do not lighten at the same time as they color. They *add* color. Usually the directions will specify that you shampoo your hair, dry it, then apply the tint which usually gives you guaranteed 100 per cent coverage.

While you can usually use tints safely yourself, they are probably best done professionally as it requires some judgment to choose the right one to use.

TWO-STEP COLORING: If you want your hair dramatically lighter—to go, for example, from medium brown to light ash blond—you must use a two-step coloring process. In other words, you must first bleach or decolorize the hair, and then tint it or tone it to the desired shade.

I implore you not to take on a two-process coloring job at home. It is just too complicated and hazardous. If your time or economic situation precludes going to an expert, then you should stick to a more simple process.

And never try for very exaggerated changes. Too many things can go wrong. Going from almost black hair, for instance, to ash blond is possible but it is not a good idea. The very lightest to which black hair can be changed without risking damage is light red. Any more and you may lose your hair altogether.

When you color your hair, particularly for the first time, and you are making a fairly drastic change (more than three or four shades), it works best if you apply the product to the ends of the hair first and work up to the roots. This is because the roots always color faster, as the natural warmth of the body activates the chemicals.

After a coloring job, wait a day or so before you judge the new color. You can't really tell right away whether it's just what you want or not. The color may change just slightly as the natural oils return to your scalp, the color oxidizes, and the setting relaxes. And don't judge it by the fluorescent light often used in bathrooms or beauty salons. The color will look quite different in natural or incandescent light.

Frosting or Streaking

This is when you lighten only some strands of hair here and there, giving a much lighter, brighter and sunnier look without going all the way. Streaking gives an effect of lightness without the headaches of overall coloring. It is especially effective for fading blondes, graying hair, red hair or light brown hair, but I happen to loathe streaks on dark hair because it is too stark a contrast and ends up looking hard and tough. (However, in the salon we often do take shampoo-in tint two or three shades lighter than the natural dark hair and streak the hair with that, giving very subtle highlights.)

There are frosting kits to be used at home, usually including a perforated cap through which the strands to be lightened are pulled. These can be quite successful the first time. But after that, better go to a colorist or you can end up with checkerboard hair.

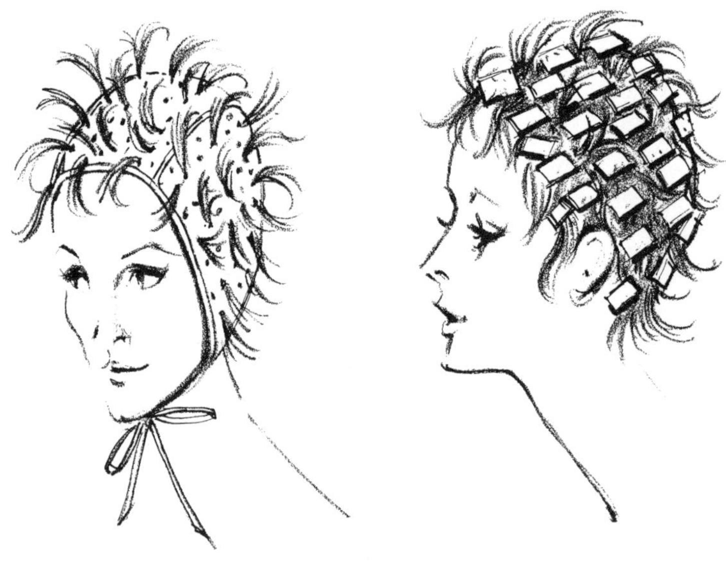

I think even the colorists should use the aluminum-foil method rather than the cap. With the foil, you pick out the strands you want to bleach and apply the chemicals to just those strands. Then you wrap them in foil to keep them separate and the product from running or getting into the hair you don't want lighter. With the cap, it is much harder to judge what hair to pull out. You may, the second time around, rebleach the same strand again, or miss the roots which need to be made lighter.

An advantage of streaking is that the hair does not have to be constantly touched up because, as it grows, the line of demarcation between the lightened hair and the natural hair is not so obvious. It should be retouched every eight to twelve weeks, depending on how fast your hair grows and how much of a contrast the frosting is. It will need retouching only at the roots where the hair has grown out. If you keep frosting all over the head, redoing the whole strands, you will eventually end up with a total color or you will be rebleaching the same hair over and over again—with all the problems that overbleaching brings.

If your streaks get too brassy or yellow from oxidation tone them down with a *temporary* rinse in a silvery or ashy shade. Don't do this with a shampoo-in color as the rest of your hair will then be permanently affected.

You can have your hair tinted or dyed over the frosting if you want to get rid of the frosting. (Occasionally some hair has been so decolorized that it doesn't accept the color easily. Professional colorists find a way out of this by using "fillers," which help the overporous hair to accept a new color.)

Bleaching can be done too, but it must be done carefully by a professional, because the hair already lightened by the frosting may now get overbleached and become fragile.

It's quite possible, if you have tinted or bleached your hair a solid color, to add highlights by streaking or frosting, though it must, obviously, be done very carefully. For example, if your hair is over 50 per cent gray you can't get a blond look by merely frosting. You must tint it a light brown or blond, and then frost it one or two shades lighter. Frosting over color is what's done, of course, when you want tone-on-tone hair. I like it much better than a solid color, but it must be done by an adept professional.

P.S. Streaking, frosting, highlighting, shading, tipping and lacing are all basically the same thing.

Reverse Frosting

This is the same process as frosting—but instead of decolorizing or lightening strands of hair, you tint them a shade or two darker with a color. We use this when we want very subtle coloring, which you can barely notice but will make the hair more interesting. Young women who don't want to look as if they have done anything to their hair and don't want allover color or real streaks, but merely a lift for dull hair, often like reverse frosting.

Or it can be used as a color correction for overfrosted hair to give more of a color to hair that's too blond.

Or if you've had a frosting and you don't like it, you can reverse-frost the streaks close to your own shade.

Reverse frosting is especially useful for women whose hair is quite gray, over 75 per cent gray, and who don't want overall color. Frosting won't work for them because the gray sections will not turn blond from a bleach. In this case, they can tint some strands of hair with a color closely matching their own original shade, giving the effect of that shade without moving on to allover color.

Reverse frosting is usually done with a permanent tint. I don't suggest you do it yourself.

Lighteners or Highlighters

There are lots of products on the market today which are known as lighteners—just wash them or brush them or spray them into your hair, and it will turn a little bit lighter. Maybe you think you can do this and then it will fade away or you can wash it out and your hair will go back to its natural color. No such thing. Lighteners—anything at all that lightens your hair—are bleaches. They may be very mild, not very concentrated, but they are still bleaches.

Again I have to tell you: I don't care what the product sounds like, what you think you are doing or not doing, there is no way to lighten your hair without its being a bleaching process. There is no such thing as a non-permanent lightener. Your hair, even if it's only a shade or two different, is forever lighter until it grows out.

If that's what you want, fine. But you should know just what you are doing.

A problem with lighteners, as with any other permanent bleach or color, is that the first time you use it you will get whatever action is built into it, and it will probably come out fine. But if you apply it again to the very same hair you've already used it on, you will be bleaching the hair another shade lighter. And now the roots won't match the ends. If you want to keep using the product, use it as a touch-up for the roots after the first time.

Of course, an old-fashioned way to lighten your hair a bit is to squeeze the juice of a lemon over your head and sit in the sun for a while. This works. And *it's* permanent too. It often, however, makes the hair quite dry and brittle.

Touch-Ups

If you bleach or color your hair with permanent coloring you must touch up the roots every three or four weeks because, as the hair grows out, it will be your old natural color. If you colored it yourself you probably just poured the solution over your hair, getting an overall effect. Well, the second time you can't just pour it on because you are then coloring two different kinds of hair—hair that was previously colored and hair that has grown out. And you'll get two different results. The important thing to know about touch-ups is that you must be most careful to work only on the grown-out hair, not on the previously tinted or bleached hair. And you must leave it on this grown-out hair the exact amount of time you left it on for the original job so that it will be the same color.

Watch that the product doesn't run or drip down. If you overlap—that means allowing the product to touch previously tinted or bleached hair—you will get dark bands of color where you've applied the tint twice, or if you are bleaching, you will find that hair previously bleached will be much lighter than the roots. Besides, you are weakening the hair with the constant chemical action. Overbleached hair becomes brittle and dry and strawlike. Overtinted hair becomes discolored and dull and dry.

Some products come in a bottle with a special tip for touch-ups. But I think it's too easy to let too much pour out this way. It really depends on you—some people are terribly careful; others are sloppy. Safer to use is a cotton swab or a touch-up brush.

Section off the hair so that the parts reveal the grown-out roots. Apply the solution only to them, section by section, following the directions given by the manufacturer.

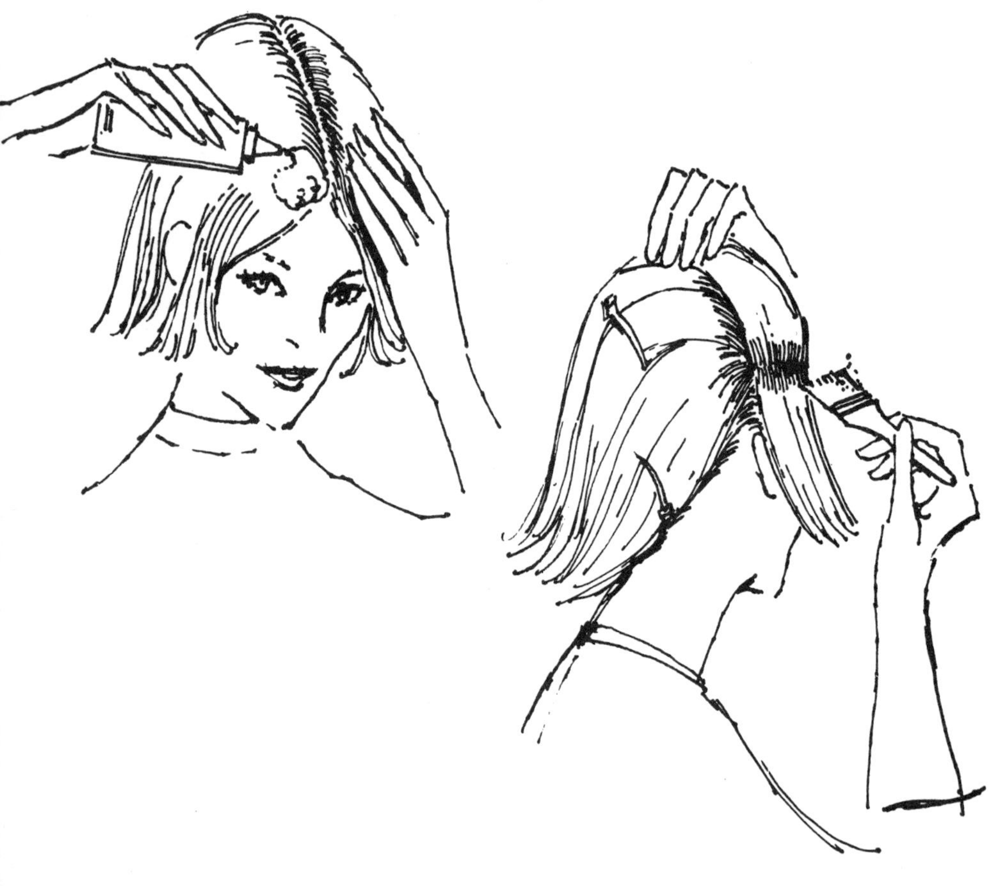

Because your hair oxidizes between colorings, after you've finished the touch-up and are the right shade, pour a little shampoo into a small amount of the leftover coloring product and quickly wash it into your hair. Then rinse it out thoroughly. This will refresh the color of the entire head of hair without making it darker than your freshly touched-up roots.

Do this refreshing if you use a shampoo tint or a tint. Do *not* do it when you are bleaching.

By the way, this will help take tint off your scalp or from around the hairline. If you still have a tinted skin, use some of the coloring agent itself to remove it.

Patch Test

Before you use a bleaching or tinting product on your hair, you must make a patch test to see if you are hypersensitive or allergic to it. If you've never used color before, if you have sensitive skin, if you're using a new product, this is especially important. But I recommend you do it every time because a change in your body chemistry may make you sensitive to a product even though you have used it for years.

You will find directions for the patch test in every package of coloring you buy. Follow them carefully. The idea is to apply a bit of the coloring product to a small patch of skin, about an inch in diameter, behind your ear or on the back of your neck or the inside of your elbow. Leave it there untouched for twenty-four hours. If no itching, redness, scaliness, irritation or moisture develops, it's probably safe for you to proceed.

Strand Test

To be sure you have chosen the right color for you, and to test the amount of time it takes to achieve it, make a strand test before you color your entire head. Do this if it's the first time you've used color or if you're using a new color. Prepare a small amount of the solution exactly as the directions tell you (again, they will be given in the package). Apply it, as suggested, to a strand of hair in the back near your ear where it won't show. Leave it the specified length of time and then check to see if the color is what you want. If it isn't leave it, and check it out at intervals, keeping careful record of the number of minutes it is left on. When you've got what you want, and you know the exact timing, go ahead with the job.

If you've made the strand test on a fair amount of hair be sure you don't color this piece again when you do the rest of the job.

Color Correction

Suppose you color your hair and you end up with something you hate. What can you do? That depends on a lot of things. Temporary coloring will, obviously, wash right out. Semi-permanent coloring will fade away, though there may be some permanent effects until your hair grows out. But permanent coloring presents sometimes insurmountable problems.

You can always make your hair darker and deeper than the color you've got and you don't like. Or you can strip the color away (bleaching) and start all over. I'm not even going to tell you how to do this because color correction is something that has to be done by an expert colorist. If you're at this deplorable point, you're there because you didn't understand what you were doing to begin with. It's time to seek the expert's advice. As I've said, sometimes if your hair is really an unhealthy mess, you're going to have to leave it alone and let it grow out.

Sometimes using a temporary rinse after every shampoo will help until your hair grows out. Or perhaps your colorist can dye your hair close to your own natural color. There really is no such thing as dyeing it its own natural color though you can come pretty close. But the very same color? It's a fantasy. And it will always change somewhat when the sun and air hit it, turning it perhaps a bit redder or lighter.

Unwanted red or gold or brassy highlights can sometimes be toned down by using a "drabber" or toner. Again go to a professional. If you keep pouring one thing after another on your head, your problems will become worse and worse.

When Not to Color

If your hair is in good condition it is usually safe to color it no matter what the texture. But if it is extremely thin or falling out, or in poor shape from oversunning, or it's been weakened by previous processes (straightening, permanenting, coloring), don't try it. Or, at least, follow the advice of an expert colorist. Never do more than one thing to your hair at once. Wait at least two weeks after a permanent to have a coloring job, and at least a month after a straightening. I prefer you don't do it at all.

Do not use coloring products—or any other chemicals—if the scalp shows any signs of irritation or eruption.

Care of Colored or Bleached Hair

Since hair coloring is chemically induced, your hair will need more careful attention than natural hair. The most important thing to consider when you color (or bleach) your hair is that because this is a chemical process it is often the *only* chemical process your hair can take. Generally speaking, you should not straighten your hair if you're going to color it, and you should not color it if you are going to straighten it. You should not permanent your hair if you're going to color it, and you should not color it if you're going to permanent it. I know there are many people who do more than one thing to their hair at once but evidently they have the texture or the amount of hair on which it works. It may not work on yours and it could lead to disaster.

If you insist on doing two chemical processes on the very same hair, wait, as I've said, at least two weeks after the first one to do the second. Never do them both on the same day. And it's best to do the coloring last. Make it no more than a one-step coloring. I'd strongly suggest that you have it done by an expert, or at least get the opinion of one before you do such a drastic thing.

Just realize that your hair is *not* going to stay on your head if you put it through one strenuous thing after another. If you've got kinky hair and you want straight hair, you may have to have straight hair that is a color you don't like. You may have to make a choice between tinting and straightening if you want to have something that has some resemblance to real hair. Women often come into my salon after they've done all sorts of horrible things to their hair and I recoil in horror. I want to run from it rather than work with it. And you can be assured that other people, especially men, feel the same way.

When you have colored your hair, you must protect it from sun, salt water, chlorine. All colored hair oxidizes and changes color as the days go by, but these things will speed up the procedure. Too much sun will turn your hair some really strange colors. If you're going to be outdoors for very long, always cover your head with a brimmed hat or a scarf. After swimming, always give your hair a good rinsing or a shampoo. Swim caps never keep the water out, so don't count on them.

Wash your tinted hair with a shampoo which is explicitly labeled for tinted and/or bleached hair. Never use very hot water; keep it lukewarm.

Condition your hair regularly, every shampoo. The coloring tends to dry and coarsen your hair and make it more porous. The conditioner will help to keep it feeling and looking better. You may want to use a product which combines shampoo with conditioner, but be sure it's designed for tinted hair.

After the shampoo, if your hair tangles, use a cream rinse to make it easier to comb when it's wet. Keep in mind, of course, that the cream rinse will soften your hair too. So, if yours is fine or limp to start with skip the cream rinse. Or rinse it out very, very thoroughly.

Don't use a brush on your wet hair. Always comb it instead, using a wide-toothed comb that won't pull your hair out. Gently comb through until all the tangles are gone. When the hair is dry, it may be brushed—but always gently.

When you roll your hair up, be careful to avoid too much tension on the rollers, and dry the hair under a warm dryer, never a hot one. Too much heat of any kind is not good for color-treated hair, so, even if you like the convenience of heated rollers, don't use them too often and then take them out after five minutes.

What I'm really saying is that color-treated hair is necessarily weakened by the chemical process—treat it with the utmost care to prevent any real damage!

Going Gray

When you start getting gray hair, you have to make a decision. Are you or are you not going to color your hair? It's an important decision and you should give it serious thought.

Gray hair isn't truly gray. It is hair that has lost its pigment and so becomes white or transparent. It usually starts appearing at the hairline, then spreads to the back. The white hairs blend with the darker hair and give an illusion of gray. These hairs tend to be quite coarse, and if in its original color the hair had a rather fine texture, you may find it's now more difficult to work with. Try using a stronger setting lotion.

Not only have the individual gray hairs lost their color pigment, but the color of the rest of your hair often fades too. The usual result after a while is a rather drab look. This isn't true of some people. Some look marvelous in their gray hair, especially brunettes whose own original color is strong enough to contrast with the gray. Many of my most attractive clients nurture their gray hair and wouldn't think of changing it. If your hair is an attractive color and it looks good on you, by all means leave it alone. Unfortunately, particularly in this country, gray hair is often considered a sign of old age or almost a disfigurement. But I think it depends very much on the individual. I've seen young women with really white hair who

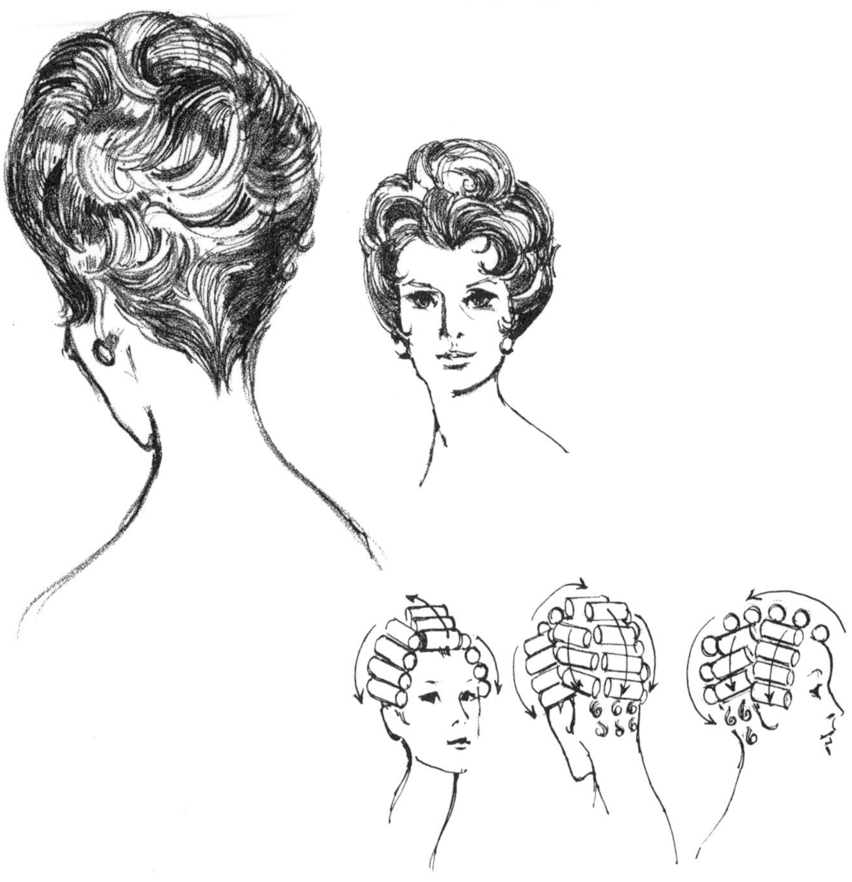

look beautiful and it would be a form of insanity to change the color.

Really black hair often goes gray very prettily; so does strong red or very blond. In other words, graying is often attractive on people with definite hair color. On not-so-definitive colors, it can be drab and dull.

Your skin tone makes a difference, too. Sallow-complexioned women usually look terrible with gray, while those with very dark or very light skins may look great. So don't consider your age in your big decision—just decide whether or not the gray hair is becoming to you. And learn how to take care of it.

You must always keep gray hair exceedingly clean for it to look beautiful. And it can because it tends to be shinier than other colors. There are a number of special products for your new hair—shampoos, conditioners, sprays, even permanent-wave lotions. Try these and see if they don't help to keep it in good condition. Remember that, just like a blonde, you must protect your hair from too much sun and salt water and other things that will tend to discolor it.

Sometimes certain vitamins, as well as perspiration, body acids, air pollution, etc., will give gray hair yellow streaks. Find a rinse designed for just this problem and you'll wonder where the yellow went.

Gray hair sometimes becomes very dry, and though this may seem a blessing if you've always had an oily scalp, it will make the hair look dull and lifeless and maybe frizzy. So keep it conditioned, brush it thoroughly every day and massage your scalp frequently.

Watch your makeup. Avoid, at any cost, any hint of sallowness. Your complexion should have a pinky quality rather than a beige or yellow. Wear bright—never dark—lipsticks and stay away from excess eye makeup which will make you look hard. If you are a mature person, I suggest eliminating powder altogether from your makeup. I think it's disastrous to an older skin, bringing out all the little lines. Just use a moisturizer and a subtle pinky-toned base on your face and neck. I'd skip the gleamers or highlighters too—they're better for the kids. Often, I think, women over sixty or so look better without any makeup at all—just as very young girls do.

One rule in my mind for gray hair is not to wear it very curly. Like blond hair, it has a tendency to show the curl too much and looks dry and frizzy as well as aging. Choose a style with curve and shape but no little curls. If you're young, long and swingy gray hair is fine. If you are older, it's far better to have a more contained hair style or a length that doesn't drag the lines of the face down—a shorter style or perhaps long hair worn up is the best solution.

What if your gray hair does nothing for you? Or, as it's busily turning gray, it develops a drab mousy shade? Then, by all means, color it. Today you can be any other color you prefer.

Now you have another decision to make. Do you want shading

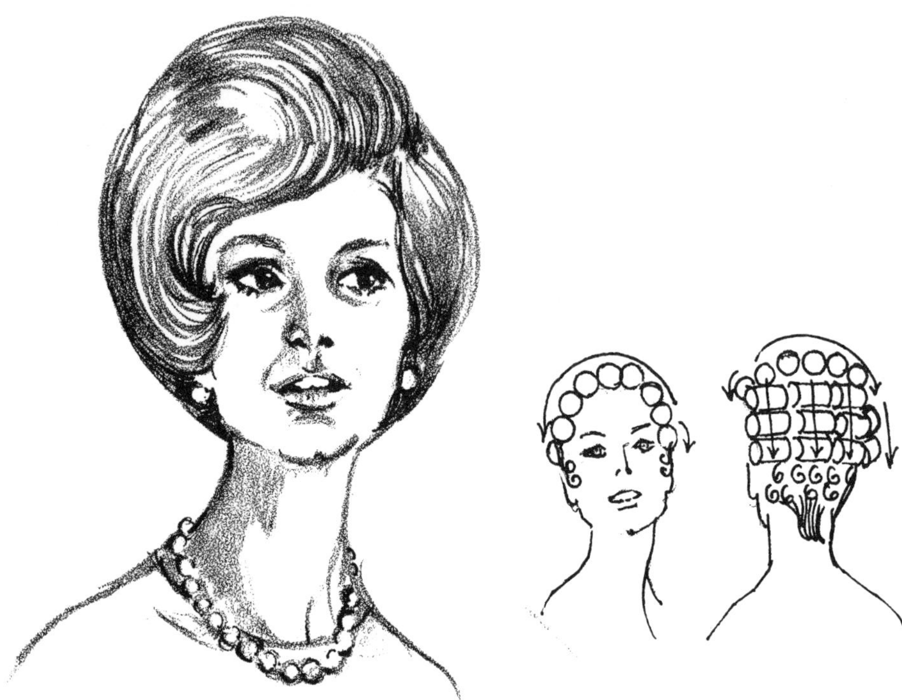

or an allover new color? I think it depends on the basic color of your hair. If it's very dark, or if it leans toward red or gold, then usually a one-process color is best, perhaps close to your own color, but always, I believe, a shade lighter. As you move into the really definite red shades, I think the place to go is a matching of your own color, but again just a little lighter. If your hair is an ashy tone, particularly a medium brown or blond which tends to become dreary as it fades, then shading (frosting, highlighting, streaking—it's all the same thing) is probably best. I'm talking about subtle shading, not zebra stripes. This means lightening strands of hair all over the head, but especially around the face. (See above.)

If your hair is too gray for shading—more than 75 per cent gray—then the route to go may be reverse frosting. (See above.)

If you are going to tint your hair an overall color, never use a coloring agent the same shade as your own hair. Always go one or two shades lighter because the very same color will make your hair look darker, denser and therefore harder. As one gets older, it's always wiser anyway to choose a lighter shade. As far as I'm concerned that's a flat rule, no matter what your basic color is. That's because your skin tone also tends to become paler along with the gray hair. This is true for Caucasian Anglo-Saxon skin colorings. Oriental, Latin and black women are often able to stay with their original dark hair and look good.

A temporary or semi-permanent color won't lighten your hair. If you want it lighter you will have to use a permanent color—either a shampoo-in product that will lighten up to about three shades or a double-process color, first bleaching and then coloring.

Occasionally the gray or white hairs do not hold color very well and it fades away, especially around the hairline. You can overcome this by an old-fashioned technique called prebleaching. If you go to a hairdresser (and I suggest you do), he will know exactly what I am talking about. If you do your own coloring, take one ounce of peroxide and two drops of 2 or 3 per cent ammonia from the *drugstore,* not the supermarket, and mix them together. Brush this on the white hair and leave it in for fifteen minutes. Wash it out and then proceed with your tint. You can, of course, also use any pure bleaching product made for hair and achieve the same thing. What you are doing is presoftening the outer cuticle of the hair, allowing it to receive and hold the color of the tint more efficiently. One caution: Do not, when you do touch-ups, overlap either the prebleaching or the tinting.

Going Black

Most of the black hair colors that were used for many years were very hard and unreal. Today, however, there is a range of darkest browns to blue blacks that produce very pretty tinted black hair—for some people. I feel, for the most part, that only people who were born with truly black hair come close to looking at all real when they use a black color. And I do think that as one grows older, somewhat lighter shades are more flattering and less aging. There are exceptions to all things, though, and I can think of several famous "beauties" who are today in their sixties, who dye their hair black and look rather startling and certainly individual. Maybe you have this kind of definitive look, but don't let your mirror lie to you.

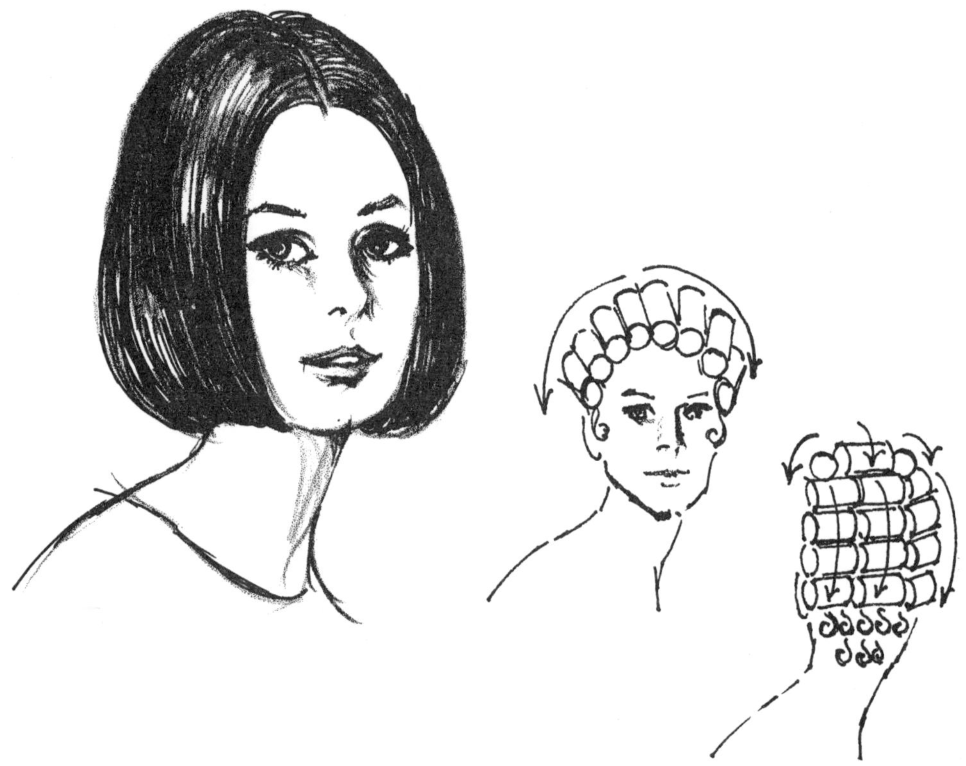

As with all other hair coloring, black looks best if it is shaded; in other words, if it is not all one solid color.

If you have naturally black or almost black hair and want to lighten it keep in mind that it cannot be lightened too much without seriously damaging it. The lightest it can become without danger is a light red.

Going Blond

Americans have always worshiped blond hair. I don't know why, but blond hair and blue eyes, the Anglo-Saxon look, is what women have always wanted. Well, they can't turn their brown eyes into blue, but it is quite possible to become a blonde. I want to warn you, however: There are lots of people who shouldn't be blondes. Many women look terrible in light hair, especially if they have dark or even faintly sallow complexions. It's time we got over this silly thing anyway—dark hair can be beautiful. It seems to me that anyone who has brunette coloring ought to give it a second thought before becoming a blonde.

Making the decision to be a blonde is a serious one and shouldn't be done as a whim, particularly if you have never done anything to your hair before. It's a big step. You needn't fear it, but you should know what you are doing and why. If you're seventeen years old,

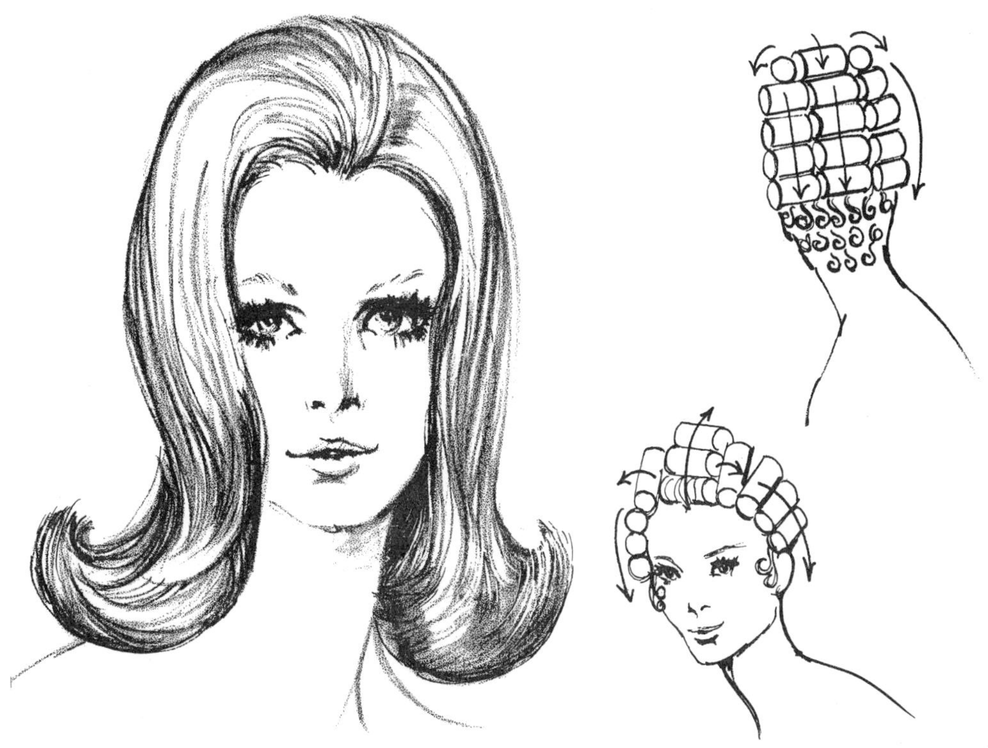

you can do almost anything and get away with it. If you're thirty or more you must be more careful because you can achieve a toughness, a hardness that is quite unattractive.

First, figure out *why* you want to be a blonde. Then, should you? Is it the most flattering thing you can do? Will your coloring take it? Most important, are you willing to maintain it? You must touch it up—there's nothing worse than blond hair with dark roots. You should have the job done professionally and then be careful not to wreck your hair by constant overlapping and overbleaching.

Now, if I've thoroughly frightened you, as I intended to do, do you still want blond hair? Fine.

I recommend it for women who have blond skin coloring though their natural hair coloring may be dark. Or for those who have blond hair that's beginning to darken, fade or go gray. Some women whose dark hair is going gray will look better blond than with their original dark color.

I don't understand some blond hair colors—the phony colors, the startling ones, the dead ones that don't reflect light. I like warm blond coloring. The ideal, I think, is almost a champagne color, a childlike color. It's real, it has life and it reflects light.

There are different kinds of blondes—I think of them as "hot" blondes and "cool" blondes. Compare Madeleine Carroll to Jean Harlow, for example. Or Eva Marie Saint to Marilyn Monroe. Dina Merrill to Jayne Mansfield. Each is (or was) a blonde, but what a difference! The definitive coloring the hair gives you has to establish you as a type. Which will you be, and is that what you're after? I don't think blondes necessarily have more fun than brunettes, but they will if they *think* they're going to.

Blond colors are four types: ash, which has no red or gold in it; golden blond, which has golden highlights; red blond, a warmer color with red highlights; and silver blond, a very pale, almost colorless shade. Which to choose depends not only on your preferences but on your skin tone. If you have a sallow or yellow complexion avoid gold shades and pick an ashy color. Better still, choose a brown color! If you have a ruddy complexion you'll look best in an ash shade. The redder tones will bring out the red in your skin. You'll have to try on wigs in different shades to be sure which is best for you.

Blond hair coloring is much better looking if it is many different shades carefully blended together, perhaps with the lightest shade right around the face.

Your hair will probably tend to become brassy from oxidation after a while. You can use a temporary drabber rinse. Better still, have the hairdresser tone it down.

Blond hair usually looks best in a simple, uncomplicated line because, like any light color, it shows every turn and curl very distinctly. Too much curl often looks frizzy.

Real Red Hair

Naturally red hair is glorious—usually. Ranging all the way from dark auburn to titian (reddish blond), it can give a woman a distinctive, flattering frame for her face. Of course, there are some shades of natural red that I think are awful. Some look angry, even "sore." If that's the case I suggest softening it by adding color to it or taking some out. Sometimes streaking, producing variations in shading, can turn a sorehead into a beauty.

Natural red hair, for some reason, always tends to be coarse rather than fine. It's strong hair. It's usually wavy rather than straight. And it's usually dry rather than oily. It often goes with very pale skin and a tendency toward freckles. I think pale skin and freckles are quite beautiful and you'd better think so too, because there's nothing to be done about them. If you've got them, you've got them.

Most redheads go gray very nicely and don't have to think of tinting their hair for a long, long time. The hair when graying seems to be shinier and more full of life than other colors. When it goes too gray to suit you, I'd suggest coloring it the same color it was originally, but perhaps a shade or two lighter.

Red hair gives such a definitive look to a person that, like very blond or very gray hair, it shouldn't be overly curled. Every line, every turn, every curve show on this coloring. So avoid frizziness at all costs. If your hair is more than wavy a slight straightening or relaxation of the curl might be in order.

Your hair should never be set in a stiff, immobile style which requires an overdose of hair spray. Like a blonde's hair, your hair has to be very free or it will get a hard look to it.

It's best, I've found, always to tone down or soften red hair. Be careful of the colors you wear. Pastels or the subtler shades will play up your hair rather than fight with it or detract from it. And be especially careful of your lipstick—sometimes you see a redhead wearing lipstick that's absolutely frightening. If your hair is orangey red, it's logical for you to wear coral lipstick. If it's a bluer tone, avoid the corals and wear a clear red or a red with blue in it.

Going Red

When I was just starting out as a hairdresser, it wasn't easy to get a good red hair color. The colorist in my salon used to use Mercurochrome to do the job. Today there's a vast range of red colorings, both in single-process and double-process procedures. And red is beautiful.

Red hair ranges from strawberry blond to auburn, but I lean toward the tones that are bright pinky or orangey rather than the purple, almost plum colors. And I like to see shading, particularly around the hairline, to make it look more natural. Just think of Lucille Ball or Arlene Dahl, both of whom have made their hair redder than it was by nature, and shaded throughout. It looks great. We made Mia Farrow a redhead for her part in *John and Mary*. I think it was very pretty.

Actually, we all have red hair. Everyone's hair goes through a red stage before it's completely decolorized in bleaching. And more and more women are deciding to let some of that red work for them. For example, a person with drab brown hair can have some of the color removed to let the red come through, making her look alive, rather than have her hair completely stripped and then tinted to make it a couple of shades lighter. Why not have a little red instead of taking such a big step? It is a one-process job and so, of course, it's healthier and easier on the hair, less expensive and time consuming, and much simpler to do at home.

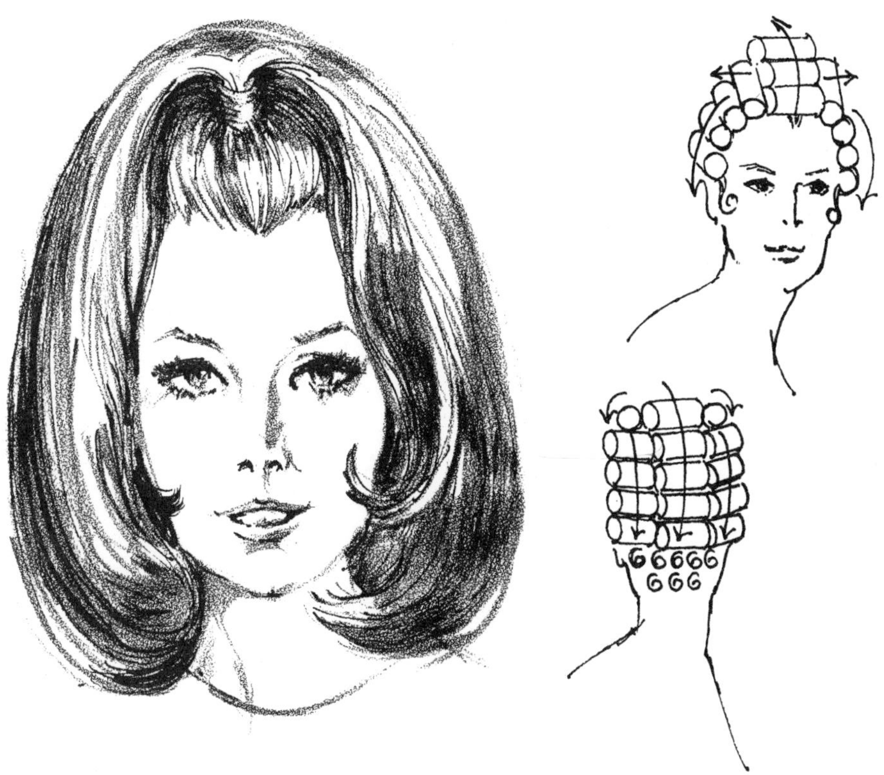

If you're looking for really red, though, you must get it the hard way. Because red hair is difficult for a lot of people to wear (sometimes even if it's natural), you should give the idea some serious consideration. If you have even a hint of a sallow complexion avoid it. Try on some wigs first to see how you'll look.

When you have tinted red hair, always use the shampoo made for tinted hair as this doesn't have a caustic stripping action others may have. Condition your hair regularly. Between touch-ups, it's quite easy to refresh your color with a light rinse.

Chapter 8

PERMANENTS AND STRAIGHTENING

If you've got straight hair that won't keep a curl or curly hair that refuses to relax—and you don't like it that way—you can change it by having a permanent wave or a straightening. The procedures

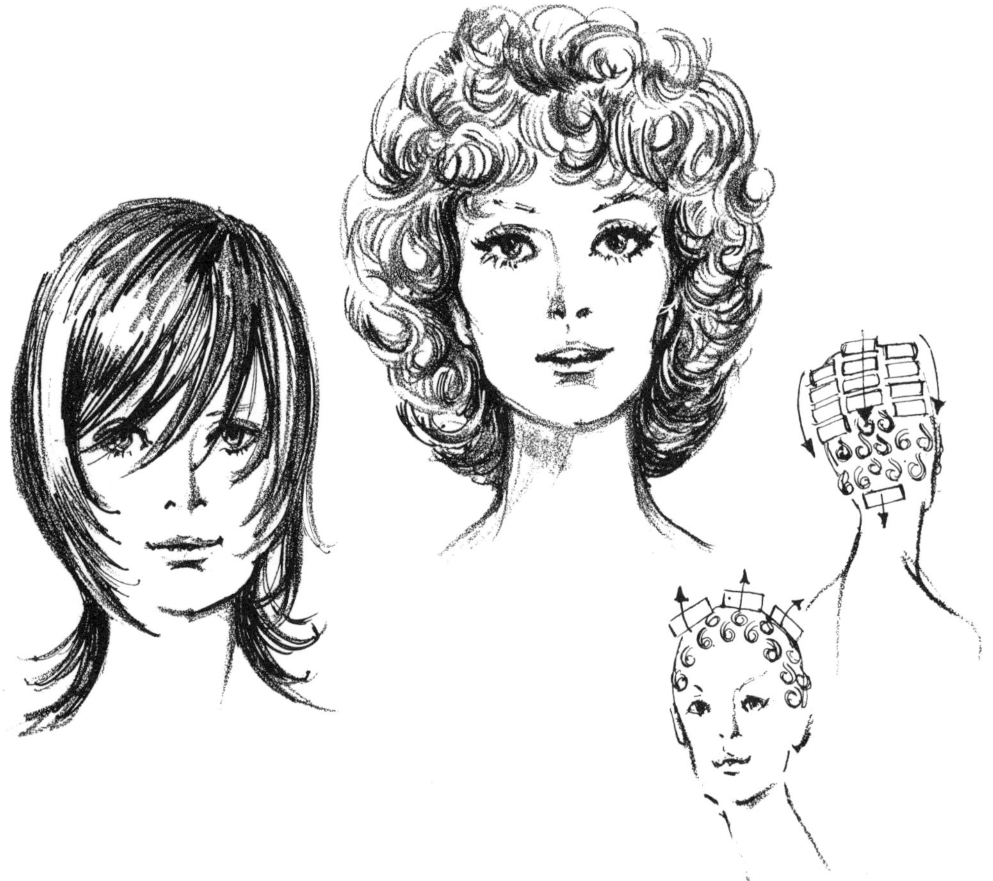

are much the same, softening the outer layer or cuticle of the hair so that it takes on the shape it's given, then neutralizing it to "fix" it permanently.

I'm not trying to drum up business, but I do feel that both permanents and straightenings are best done by professionals. Lots of women give themselves good permanents at home, but they're the people who follow directions to the letter, or have a friend who's very handy with permanent-wave rods, have strong, healthy hair that hasn't been mistreated, and know just what they want.

Straightening is another story. This, I feel, must never be done at home because it can cause almost irreparable damage to the hair.

Permanents

The usual reason for having a permanent wave is to give longer lasting results from a setting, as well as body to the hair. Some hair is so fine or so straight or so limp that it doesn't hold a set more than a day or two. A permanent can give it more substance and/or curl. A "body wave," which is a permanent but done on larger rods, merely gives the hair more bulk and holding power and usually a very slight wave pattern. A "permanent wave" gives curl or wave.

Permanents fell out of fashion quite a few years ago. It's at least a generation since women took on the "perm" as a necessity. Hair styles haven't required it and younger women just plain resisted the overly frizzed hair of their mothers and grandmothers. For many years, women planned on two permanents a year and the idea was to get that permanent as tight as possible because it was believed it lasted longer that way. I can remember almost twenty-five years ago in hairdressing school when the teachers explained to us that we should always tell the client, if the permanent came out *too* tight, "wait and see how wonderful it will look in a month." I think that's probably what finally undid permanent waving.

Just recently there's been a lot of flak about the return of the permanent wave because there's a strong trend, both in this country and in Europe, toward curlier hair. I suppose it's because there are many women who have become bored with their straight hair and because this new generation, which has never worn curly hair and never had a permanent, is enjoying the idea of a change. Maybe just the camp of it is appealing.

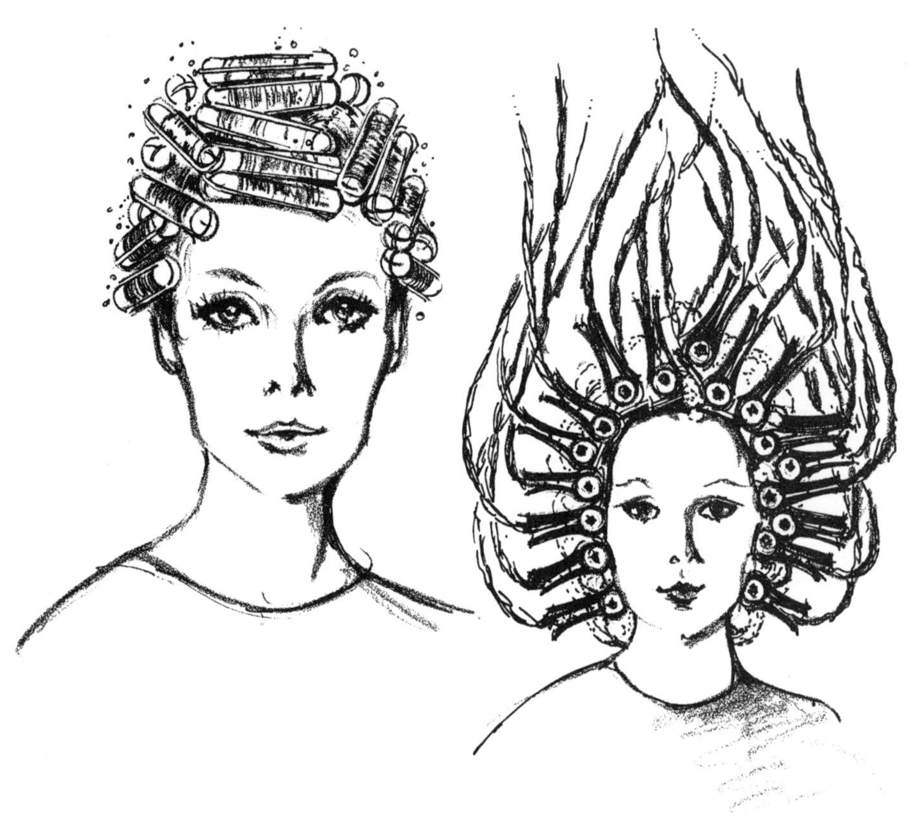

The permanent wave is about fifty years old. The first permanents in the early '20s were called spiral waves and required the hair to be wound lengthwise from the scalp out to the ends on long thin rods, then hooked up to a heat machine. Next came the croquignole wave, also using electrically induced heat, but the hair was rolled from the ends in toward the scalp.

These early-day permanents took a long time to give and were very expensive. They were also rather dangerous—there were plenty of stories about those poor souls who emerged from the beauty parlor without their hair.

Then came the machineless wave, with chemical softeners in the permanent-wave lotion, and heat induced by a chemical pad without electricity.

All of these waves worked very well in their time, especially on virgin hair. They were, however, more than a bit touchy on tinted or bleached hair. But then, far fewer people colored their hair in those days.

Early in the '40s, a revolutionary new permanent arrived on the scene. This was the "cold wave," a totally chemically induced wave requiring no heat. Though much improved, this is still what is used today.

Because I think it's always wise to know something about what is happening to you, I will try to explain as simply as possible what today's permanent waves do.

The Modern Permanent

The first step of a modern permanent is usually the application of the wave lotion which presoftens the hair. Then the hair is wound on rods. It is vital that the hair is wet through evenly with the lotion, that the winding is careful and done without tension, and that end papers are always used.

The next step is to rewet the entire wound-up head with lotion. This is called processing. What is actually happening is that the hair is being softened and the outer layer or cuticle is being, in a sense, broken down so that the hair will take on the form of the rod.

Now comes the neutralizer, a lotion which, depending on the particular product, is left in the hair or rinsed out. This replaces chemically the outer layer and locks in the wave pattern. It is the most important step. More permanent waves fail because of insufficient or careless neutralizing than anything else.

Permanents and Color

Today's permanent is generally safe on almost all kinds of hair *except* double-process bleached or tinted hair. That means hair that has been decolorized by a bleach and then has had color added, in a two-step procedure. For this, there are products especially made, and if they are administered by a careful technician, they can work very well. If not, disaster. Most hairdressers try to talk clients with double-processed color out of having a permanent. I usually do. Certainly, I would strongly recommend that you do not give yourself a home permanent with this kind of hair.

In any case, it is important that the right product is used for your particular kind of hair. If your hair has been bleached, even by a one-step process, the permanent will "take" more quickly than it would on natural hair. Any color treatment makes the hair more porous, so that it absorbs the wave lotion faster. If you permanent your own hair be sure to choose a product made for color-treated hair.

If you color your hair it is better to have the permanent between colorings, never immediately before or after, never on the same day. The permanent should come first, then the color. Wait at least two weeks.

Test Curls

A test curl, in any case, no matter what kind of hair you have, should be done before the whole head is permanented. Everybody's hair reacts differently to the chemicals. Dry or brittle or fine hair, for example, can become frizzy with the same amount of time that oily, coarse hair will become gently curled.

If you test-curl a strand of hair you can avoid overprocessing and help yourself come out with the proper amount of curl. Pretesting should always be done, whether a hairdresser gives you the permanent or you give it to yourself. Directions will be given on the package. And if you've had poor permanents in the past, make more than one test curl, trying the timing out on various sections of the head.

Helpful Hints

Always give yourself a permanent wave in normal room temperature—65° to 75°. If you have direct cold air on your head, from an air conditioner or an open window, the process will usually take longer. And if the temperature is very hot, it will be faster.

A permanent holds its tensile strength up to three or four months, depending on the texture or natural elasticity of the hair. Most hair grows about half an inch a month, so you'll need a new permanent about three times a year. It's best to have as much of the old permanent as possible cut off before a new one is given. To overlap another permanenting process over an old one is again courting trouble. Or at the very least, you will not get the best results.

Before you have a permanent, your hair should be in the best possible condition. If it isn't give yourself a few weeks of conditioning treatments before the big step. And always condition it right before the permanent.

It's quite possible to permanent only one area of the hair. For instance, the underneath hairline at the nape, which may be the straightest section of the head and won't stay curled. Or just the crown where we often do maybe ten curls to give height or lift.

Except for some very young girls who are wearing their permanented heads washed and dried and as frizzy as possible, any kind of permanent must be set. This doesn't mean it must necessarily be set in the conventional roller manner, but it has to be set somehow after a washing or a wetting if you don't want chaos on your head. Perhaps a place set or blow-dry will do it, but usually you'll need more than that, for the purpose of a permanent is to hold the line of hair so it springs back into shape with some direction from you. You cannot have the best of all possible worlds. Your permanent will help keep the set in, but for that help, you are trading something. Usually, you can't go swimming and let your hair dry in the sun; nor can you wear it in a wash-and-wear style. It's a matter of priorities.

Too Much Curl

What if you get a permanent that is too curly? How can you get rid of it? That's a tricky business. I'd suggest setting your hair on very big rollers with some strong setting lotion and controlling it that way. Never, never put any straightening chemicals on it. *Never.* This will be much too much for your hair to take.

Sometimes the curl is taken out with the very same lotion that put it there in the first place—the permanent-wave lotion. The lotion is combed through the hair until it's fairly straight, and immediately neutralized. This can be done, but I recommend you don't try it because it's asking the hair to take too much abuse. It's a double chemical treatment, like leaving the lotion on the hair twice as long as it should be left on. Besides, it is very difficult to control just how much curl you will be taking out this way—*all* the curl may come out. Unless you are desperate and willing to chance real problems, I would avoid this at all costs. Better to try to cope with the curl until it grows out and can be cut off.

Permanent or Body Wave?

The smaller the rods used in winding the hair, the curlier the wave will be. And that is the basic difference between a "permanent" and a "body wave." They are really the same thing—a body wave having a one- to two-inch wave pattern, and a permanent a half-inch to one-inch pattern.

Tell the hairdresser what you're after and then let him decide which you need. In general, hair that is long, fine and sparsely spaced could be given more substance with a permanent. Long, fine but thick hair would do better with a body wave. If you want a definite curled or waved style a permanent is the answer. If you want your hair just to stay in shape better then it's a body wave. The real control here is the size of the rod and occasionally the strength of the wave lotion. A body wave is done on very large rods, sometimes taking larger sections of hair per curler to produce the larger wave pattern. A body wave will not be excessively curly, even when it's not set.

Straightening

In most cases, if you don't like your curly hair you don't have to have it. Get it straightened.

If your hair is terribly curly or frizzy it can be a real problem unless you want to have it cut in a natural shape and use what nature presented you with. We've just come out of an era when straightening often seemed necessary to people because of the generally straight hair fashions. Now there is a small movement "back to nature," and there will probably be more women who will wear their hair natural, with whatever curl, wave or even frizz it may have, right there for all the world to see. The same may well apply to those with straight hair.

But if you find that your curly hair is a cross to bear, a situation you find too difficult to cope with, something that brings you anguish, investigate the possibility of straightening it.

In a way, straightening is a permanent in reverse. A protective cream is applied around the hairline and sometimes all over the scalp. Then the chemical solution is applied to the hair starting at the curliest area, and combed through to distribute it evenly. When enough of the curl is gone—and that is the tricky part—the solution is rinsed out and quickly neutralized. The neutralizing, an essential step, chemically sets the hair in the straight pattern, "hardens" it in a sense. It must be done carefully and thoroughly. If it's just slapped on, there will be problems.

Always go to a professional for a straightening job. Go to an ex-

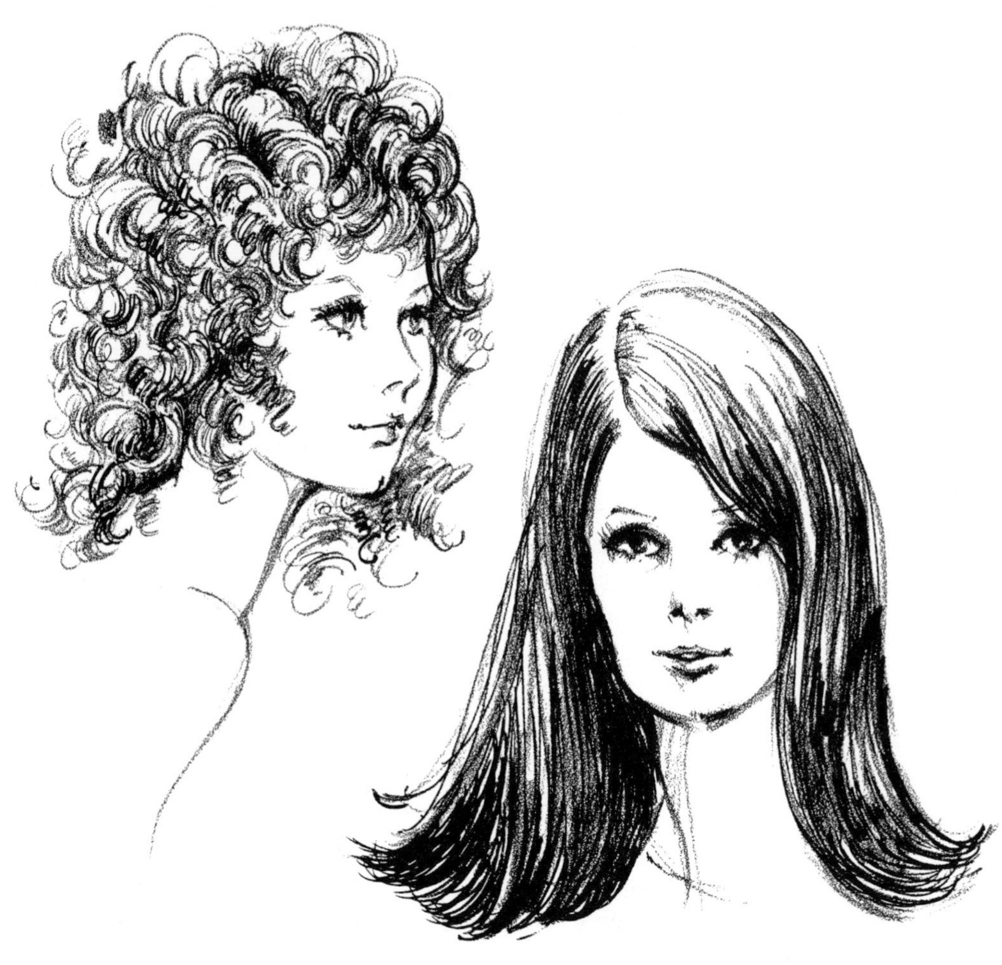

pert—there are people who specialize in it and do practically nothing else. *Never* do it yourself at home. Straightening is the toughest, most potentially damaging thing that can be done to your hair. Let me explain that statement by telling you that the straightening lotion, quite similar to permanent-wave lotion but stronger, is close in chemical content to a depilatory. It is a softener which breaks down the structure of the hair. If left on too long it will "eat" or dissolve it. If too much tension is placed on the hair while the lotion is working it can break off.

If you insist on doing the job yourself, then remember it is essential to follow the directions exactly. Although there are some good products for home use, I find that people tend not to read or follow directions. In the case of straightening, what more can I say? If you don't do it properly you may find that a wig is not only desirable but necessary because you will end up with bald spots, scabs, and clumps of hair falling into your soup.

Always make a careful strand test on a piece of hair which doesn't show to be as sure as possible of doing a successful job.

Limitations of Straightening

There are degrees of straightening. You can take a little of the curl out, some of the curl out or nearly all of the curl out. You can have only certain parts of your hair straightened. It depends on what you want and what kind of hair you have. Coarse hair is the safest to straighten because it is the strongest. Very fine hair needs more caution—you can't leave the solution on very long without ruination.

Don't ever expect to get bone-straight hair. Don't strive for luxurious flowing locks or you may be disappointed. Some hair is too curly or too fine to be made perfectly straight without danger of damage. So I suggest you try to be happy with whatever straightening you can get. You'll still probably feel you look two thousand times better with some of the kink removed.

Some women find that by straightening their hair they end up with straight but very bodiless, very limp hair. This is another reason why I strongly suggest you should never try for absolute straightness.

Sometimes the hair will straighten better the second time around. This is often true of excessively curly hair which can't be completely straightened the first time. Once it's been straightened and has grown out for six months, it may be a little easier to handle.

Very often we straighten just those parts of the hair that need it most. Some women have hair that gets very frizzy right around the face, but the curl at the ends doesn't bother them. Some women need only the crown smoothed out.

How do you know if straightening is safe for you? If your hair is natural and untouched by any chemical process it is probably safe. If it has been colored or bleached there may be a question—a big one—and only the expert can tell you the answer. Frankly I'd rather not attempt it.

If you want color then get it *after* a straightening. Sometimes you may have to make a choice of the two. Your hair may not be able to take both treatments together, even with the coloring done afterward. Never, never straighten two-process colored hair, or have a two-process color done on straightened hair.

Though I know it's often done more than that, I don't think it's advisable to have a straightening more than twice a year, preferably once at the start of the summer when your hair will normally be the curliest because of the humidity. At the end of six months, you will have about three inches of new hair to be worked on. If the straightening is done more frequently there is very little new virgin hair and overlapping is almost inevitable. Putting the strong lotion on the same hair over and over again can't be anything but bad.

Treat straightened hair with the utmost kindness. Just like bleached or tinted or permanented hair, any hair that's been chemically treated can be adversely affected by sun, salt water, chlorine. Cover it in the sun. Rinse it out after a swim. Don't put excess strain or tension on it—no heavy teasing, powerful brushing, tight ponytails, brush rollers, etc.

Once you've straightened your hair, it is straight, that's it. You can set it, but you cannot put the curl back in. Of course, as your hair grows out, the new hair will have its natural wave or curl pattern and often that pattern is so strong that it will throw even the straightened hair into a somewhat wavy look. Even if this is the case, *do not* restraighten your hair or you're courting trouble.

Chapter 9

WIGS AND HAIRPIECES

Wigs are the hats of the '70s. Like many fashion accessories, they are Instant Cinderella. They are second heads for women who have collected entire wardrobes of them. I can tell you that women are always in a hurry and it's terribly handy to be able to pop on a whole new head of hair whenever you feel like it.

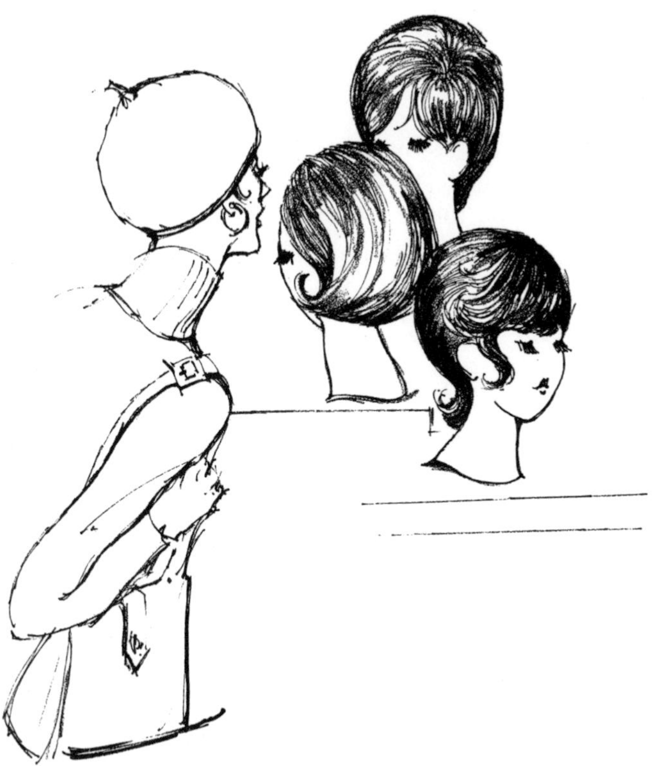

The smaller hairpieces—falls, wiglets, braids, etc.—are designed for quick-change instant hairdos using your own hair along with them. Think of them as you think of eyelashes—an accepted cosmetic, another way to change your look. Fast.

Fake hair used to be worn only out of necessity by people who were going bald. Then about 1956, a French designer showed a collection with his models wearing wigs. The idea made headlines, and before long, everyone was panting for wigs. The race was on. More and more fake hair was made and sold, with almost a half billion dollars in sales in the United States alone in 1971.

The first fashion hairpieces were made of real human hair. Many still are, but there are now some marvelous synthetic fibers which really look like hair, are less expensive and perform very well.

Wigs and the smaller hairpieces aren't as "wiggy" as they once were. They can look very real if you choose carefully. They are comfortable, lightweight and can radically change your look in a matter of seconds—from straight to curly, curly to straight, from blond to red or black, short to long—without having to fuss with your own hair. And they're a great convenience for anyone who has any of the basic hair complaints—hair that's fine, thin, oily, bodiless, etc.—which means your hair doesn't look good very much of the time.

There is an enormous range in prices for false hair. One lady wrote to me saying she'd read that one of my clients had purchased a fall of hair from me for $1,100. She couldn't imagine what would make anything so expensive when there were falls available for $30—or even $15.

The client she had read about had bought a fall which was thirty-six inches long, very pale blond with paler highlights. It was very thick, custom-blended, handmade and top-quality European hair. All of which made it cost a lot of money. If it had been made of top-quality European hair but shorter, a darker color and machine-made, it would have cost considerably less. Even less if it were made from the more plentiful Oriental hair which is rarely made to order or custom-blended. And if it had been synthetic it would have been an entirely different story. Like so many other things, you get what you pay for. I don't think anybody could argue the point that a beautiful, handmade, first-quality European-hair wig or hairpiece is the best. However, at this point in time, this is a very expensive proposition because of the high costs of both the labor and the hair.

But the synthetic hairpieces are terrific, and we sell thousands and thousands of them. In fact, they account for more than 90 per cent of the sales today. In the last few years, the synthetics have developed into a really good product. I'm quite willing to admit that there are some awful ones around, especially the very cheap ones, but this is true also of shoes, bags, any other accessory you might buy.

I firmly believe, as more and more women find the proper wig or hairpiece for themselves and experience the convenience that it gives them, that these accessories will become a staple in every woman's wardrobe.

Real-Hair Wigs and Hairpieces

These are a serious investment, so don't just walk into a store and walk out with a human-hair wig. Go to a reputable shop and, if possible, an authority on the subject. You'll be spending a lot of money and it's important to choose carefully. Be sure the piece is well shaped and fits your head perfectly. Then have it cut to suit you by *your own hairdresser,* since he knows your look and your life style better than the stranger who sells it to you in the shop. If you can buy it from your hairdresser (and be sure he really knows what he's about on this subject), that's even better. *Never* use your own scissors on it. *A wig or hairpiece doesn't grow.*

CLEANING: You must never wash or shampoo a real-hair hairpiece, whether it's Oriental or European hair. You can irreparably damage the foundation and the hair. It must be dry-cleaned and then set and dried much like your own hair. How often to have it cleaned depends on how often you wear it and whether your head is very oily or if you perspire heavily. On the average, I suppose it could use a cleaning about every eight or ten wearings. I'd strongly advise having it serviced by a professional. You can do awful things to it yourself and professional care will make a big difference in how long it lasts.

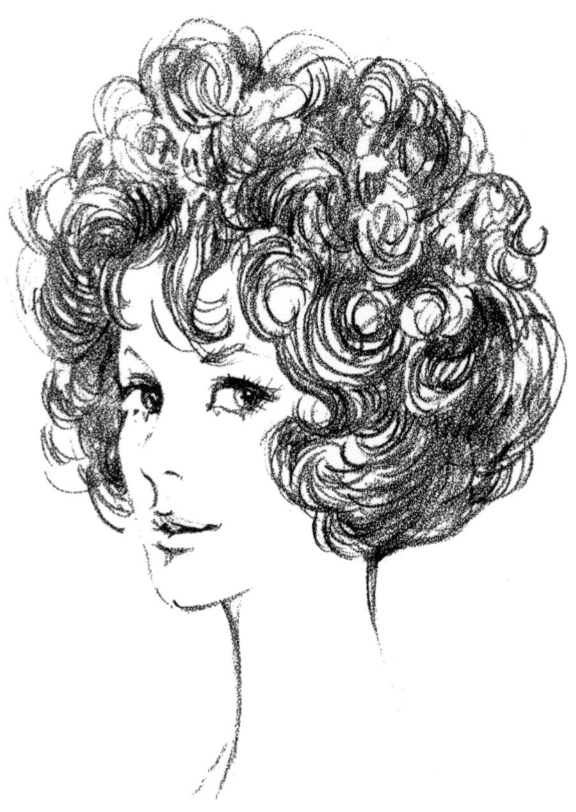

But you can clean it yourself if you use *extreme care.* There are cleaning fluids especially made for this purpose. You clean the hair by dipping it in and out of the solution, wrapping it in a towel to blot up the excess fluid, then gently combing or brushing. The hair must then be set much as you would set your own and dried.

One caution: Most of these cleaning fluids are extremely flammable and must be used in a clear open space away from heat or flame.

SETTING: To set a real-hair wig or hairpiece, pin it first to a wig block. I never use setting lotion but just lukewarm water. Be very careful not to wet the foundation and not to get the hairpiece sopping wet. The best method is to dip your comb into a glass of lukewarm water, and moisten each section as you set it. Set as you would your own hair, on rollers or in pin curls. Roll on the rollers and hold each with a large rust-proof T-pin pushed through the roller and into the wig block. For pin curls, use rust-proof clips.

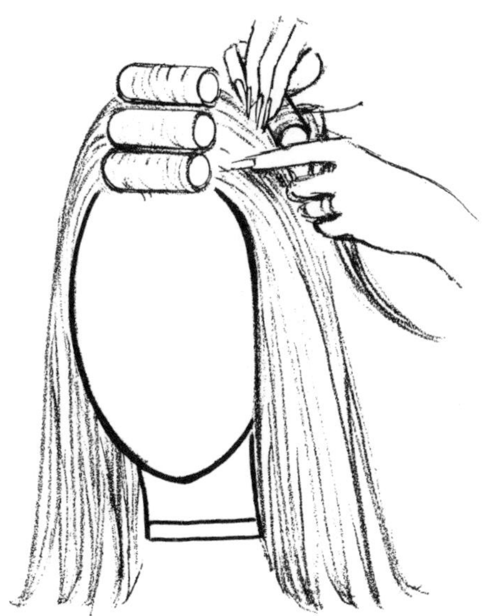

Dry under a dryer set at medium, not hot, for about a half hour. Then let it dry in the air overnight.

To comb out the set, leave the wig or hairpiece pinned to the wig block and remove the rollers or pin curls. Brush out completely. Place hair into the basic shape you want, brushing the back first, then the sides and then the top. If you need some height tease *just a little* with a gentle touch. Always brush and comb gently. Hair that you pull out won't grow back.

Try not to use hair spray on your wig. If you have to, use the absolute minimum. We use regular lacquerless, water-soluble hair spray, though there are many so-called "wig sprays" on the market today. Most of them have a lot of lanolin in them which has some validity, I suppose, though you must be extremely careful that you don't get too much on. If you do you'll have to clean the wig again because the hair will start to stick together.

CARE: Your real-hair hairpiece should be conditioned occasionally, just like your own hair, so it doesn't lose its sheen and softness. You can do it yourself if you clean your wig yourself, but again I recommend you have it done professionally.

It's wise to keep a real-hair wig pinned to a wig block and in a box. It needs air so don't cover the box tightly; just drape a scarf over the top to keep out the dust. Chiffon works beautifully. Wrapping in plastic except en route is to be avoided as the plastic will hold dampness which will eventually ruin the wig. Keep the box in a dark place because too much light will tend to oxidize the color, especially the Oriental pieces which are bleached and dyed to start with. And cover your wig when you are out in the sun to prevent a color change.

A little rain won't hurt your real-hair wig or piece, though it may make your set droop, but if you're caught in a real downpour, you should take it to a professional for a reblocking as soon as you can. Always carry a plastic rain scarf with you just in case.

COLORING: Just like your own hair, a real-hair wig can be bleached or dyed, or streaked or curled, though we often advise against it if it's a really major color change and we feel the hair can't take it. That's because if you ruin your wig it's ruined. It won't grow back again. You can destroy the hair, or all the chemicals, coloring products, and shampoos can cause the ventilated or wefted base to fall apart.

Sometimes the hairpiece will become faded or dull just through exposure and wear. If this happens, have it color-rinsed by an expert.

If it loses thickness here and there after wearing it a long time you can have new hair filled in to give it more bulk, although any handwork of this sort is now terribly expensive. Many people do this, however, as a wig can become as comfortable and as familiar as a favorite pair of shoes.

It's getting harder and much more expensive to obtain first-quality, real human hair. Make certain you know exactly what you want and, most important, that it is a design and a style you can cope with. Your "second head" shouldn't have to go to a hairdresser for a combing every time you wear it.

If you take really good care of your hairpiece it will last you a long time, depending, of course, on the wear you give it.

Occasionally, a woman will have a wig or hairpiece made from her very own hair. If her hair is very long and she decides to have it cut short, this is quite possible. We've done it for many clients. You must keep in mind that this is an expensive procedure, even though it's your own hair, because of the labor involved. And it will take from three to six weeks to make. Your hairpiece will not be as long as the cut-off hair because you have to figure that a good two to four inches will be used in the tying. So, if you cut off twelve inches, your hairpiece will be perhaps eight or nine inches long. Often the hair is good all the way down to the ends, but sometimes the ends are split or broken and may need to be trimmed off. This, too, can shorten the piece. If you haven't enough bulk for the hairpiece, though, extra hair can easily be blended into it.

Synthetic Hair

When synthetic hair first came on the scene, it was pretty horrible. It looked frankly fake and most people who wore it were better dressed for a costume party than a dinner party. It lacked movement and swing and any sense of fashion. The mass popular wig style was the short, cropped, close-to-the-nape, curly-topped wig, purchased mainly by women between thirty-five and sixty-five. The most popular hairpiece was a long, straight, too-shiny fall.

Today there are synthetic fibers that really look like hair (better than your own hair, in some cases), and there are hundreds of different styles and colors. The popular prices range from about $10 up to $60 or $70. Synthetic hairpieces can be washed like a pair of nylons. They look almost like real hair but they behave better. They aren't affected by humidity and they dry quickly. They pack in small spaces, can get caught in bad weather and fall right back into shape with a few strokes of the brush.

Synthetic hairpieces are styled by baking the forms into the fiber, giving them a permanent shape. You can't set most of them because they won't take a curl. You can't unset them because the shape won't come out—unless, of course, you use excessive heat which will ruin them in a hurry. Like most synthetic fibers, they can even melt.

The style most synthetic pieces have is the style they're always going to have—it is cooked into them. You can comb them many different ways, but you cannot change the basic form.

That's true for most of the fibers. There is, however, a new American-made fiber, which I've been working with. This not only has the ability to hold its "baked-in" setting but can also be set just as your hair might be. It has a very real hair quality to it, both in touch and look. This fiber has a set or a prestyle built into it. When it's washed it has a memory and bounces back to that style, but you can set it into something else if you want to. That is a great option.

This fiber can be set with heated curlers, but my preference is to put it up with water in rollers or pin curls, and dry it under a warm dryer. This is better for the wig and gives a better set. *Allow to cool completely before removing the rollers in order to retain the curl.* It will last about as long as a set will on your own hair. Eventually it will return to whatever style was originally baked in.

Synthetic hair can be cut, but please don't let just anyone—especially the salesgirl you buy it from—cut it for you. Take it to your hairdresser if it needs shaping and let him do it for you. Be careful with the cutting. If you cut off the curl, there's no way to put it back in permanently.

WASHING: A good brushing every few days will keep your synthetic hair fresh and clean. Wash it about every eight or ten wearings. If your head perspires a lot or is very oily, do it more often

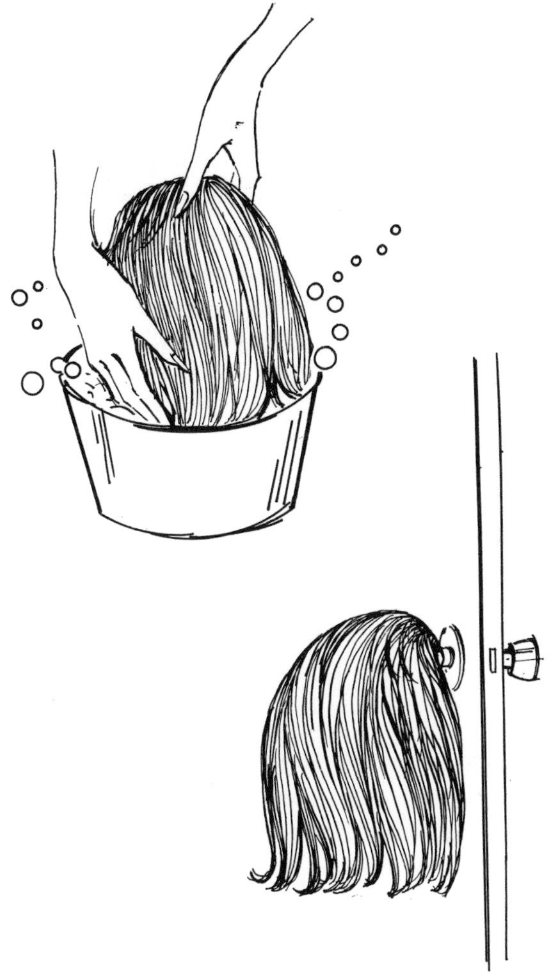

because the base will get soiled. Many manufacturers claim you can toss a synthetic hairpiece or wig into a washing machine. I guess you can, but I don't recommend it any more than I'd recommend washing your stockings that way. I prefer hand washing with a mild detergent, pure soap, shampoo or special wig wash, using cool or lukewarm water. Hot water can wreck the set. Wash it gently, dipping it in hair side first and swishing it around a few times. No rubbing, no twisting. Rinse thoroughly in cool water. If your particular wig seems to be full of static electricity, try a little fabric softener in the rinse water. Blot in a thick towel and then hang it up to dry on a doorknob or a tub faucet—away from heat.

COMBING: Don't comb or brush it while it's wet. Just let it hang there until it's completely dry. Then you can brush it and the style will fall right back into place. I recommend using a wire brush because nylon creates too much static electricity, as does a plastic comb. Always brush gently, being careful not to catch the brush bristles in the base, tearing it, or to pull any of the hairs out.

I advise never using spray on a synthetic wig or fall. It doesn't need any. If you feel you must, however, be certain to use a water-soluble spray and use it very, very lightly.

If you use hair spray you will eventually get a build-up on the hair. Because you wash it in cool water, you can't always get the spray out and it may get dry and brittle or sticky and dirty-looking.

I also recommend never teasing a synthetic hairpiece. But people do. If they do it carefully and gently it might be OK, but often they end up with a mess on their hands.

REHABILITATION: If you happen to have such a mess take it someplace where they know how to handle it. Just recently, a customer came into my salon bringing along a synthetic fall she'd purchased from us—a very expensive, handmade, custom-blended fall. It was unbelievable. She had been to the tropics, spent about five months there, used her fall constantly, sprayed it, teased it, abused it, and obviously had never washed it, combed it or brushed it. We managed to give it a thorough cleaning and softened it up some, but I assure you it will never be as good as it once was or could still have been.

Here's what to do yourself if you want to try to rejuvenate a tormented synthetic wig or hairpiece with spray build-up and snarls. First, very carefully brush it out with a wire brush, taking out all the teasing and some spray as well.

Then, in cool or just lukewarm water, using a wig shampoo or regular shampoo, let it soak at least ten minutes. Rinse thoroughly in cool water. Comb out. Feel the fibers to see if you've got them clean. If not, repeat the operation. If the hair feels stiff or there's been a lot of breakage dip it again in cool water to which you've added some cream rinse. Let it sit for five minutes. Then rinse again.

Before I leave this subject, I'd like to say once more that there is really no point in buying a pretty wig or hairpiece which looks great the way it is—it *should* or you shouldn't have bought it—and then turning it into a plastic tangle. Free, luxurious, attractive hair is not besodden with hair spray nor teased into a snarl.

COLORING: Synthetic hair cannot be bleached or dyed. There's no way. You cannot change the basic color which has been "locked in" during the manufacture of the fiber. It is possible, however, to color-rinse synthetic hair; in other words, to add a coat of color to it. When you do this, just as with real hair, you cannot go lighter. You can only go darker or brighter. You can put black rinse on a brown wig, for example. Or you can add red highlights. But you cannot lighten it or do a real permanent dye job, and you must repeat it about every four shampoos.

If you're adding color because you prefer it that's one thing. But if you're doing it because your synthetic wig has become faded or dull through wear I really think it's time to get a new one instead.

To color-rinse synthetic hair, buy a wig rinse and use it according to the directions given. Each one is different. And be sure your particular fiber can take it.

Wigs

A wig should always look better than your own hair. Otherwise, why did you buy it? That means not only buying a good-looking wig but also not teasing and combing and spraying it into an iron-clad mess so that it loses all the attractiveness of its hairlike quality.

A wig—and smaller hairpieces as well—should never look as if you walked under a tree and it fell on you. It should look as if it is your very own hair. You must choose well and then learn to use it skillfully.

The most successful wig, the easiest to cope with, has some sort of bangs so that the hairline is covered. This makes it easier to work with, though there are wigs where you can use your own hair in front (you must be more adept for these). It should have a feathery cut around the face and in the back so it won't sit woodenly on your head. Though wigs can be made to fit your own particular head, most wigs today have a one-size stretch base because they're so much easier to deal with. They fit like hats.

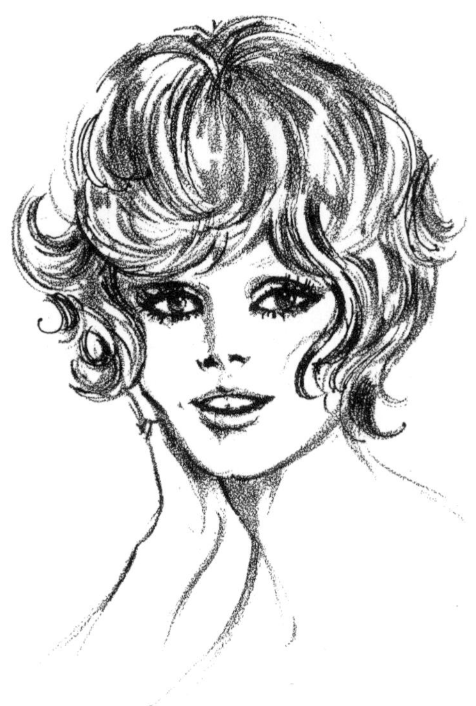

When you buy your wig, be sure it fits well and is comfortable. It is not returnable. It should go on your head easily and stay put snugly without binding. It should feel almost like you're wearing nothing.

Consider the color carefully. If you buy a wig that's drastically different in color from your own hair be sure it's really flattering to you and that you'll have the nerve to wear it. The first wig you buy will probably approximate your own color, but after that you will probably want to experiment with shades a little bit lighter or a little bit darker than your own. Always be sure that many tones of hair have been blended together to give a natural appearance—no real head of hair is all one color.

Are you a person who can carry off the fantasy of a totally different hair color or hair style than it is probable or possible your own hair could have? In other words, are you prepared to let everybody know you are wearing a wig? I don't think it matters, but it's something to think about. It's fun to have a totally new head when the mood strikes you, but it shouldn't look completely implausible. If you are a sporty, casual, natural-looking person you will not want to buy a wig that is too big or too set or too unreal. And you don't have to. There are wigs today which have a small-head, natural look in which all the style and the look come from the cut that's made in the manufacture. Unfortunately, most women choose wigs that look like the hairdos most American women still wear—set, teased, sprayed, glued and immobile. It's a pity. But you don't have to follow along. Search until you find a wig you like.

Many people worry about whether wearing a wig constantly will hurt their own hair. First of all, I don't think anyone—unless she's going bald—will wear a wig constantly. It's really an aid for the times your own hair doesn't look good. I do believe that it's healthy for the scalp to be able to "breathe" some of the time and so I would say, don't wear your wig to bed or around the house. Put it on when you're going out in public.

Used this way, a wig won't hurt your hair a bit. In fact, many women have told me their hair has vastly improved since they've been wearing a wig. That's because they've stopped doing all the terrible things they used to do to it—all the excessive teasing, spraying, dyeing, bleaching, straightening, etc. Now they leave their own hair alone and that is definitely good.

PUTTING ON A WIG: For a wig to look good, your own hair mustn't be all lumpy underneath. Nor must it creep out around the edges. It must look just as good in back as it does in front.

The best way to arrange short hair under a wig is to cover it with a cap—you can buy one or make one from an old nylon stocking—and tuck all the little ends underneath. Or just pull your hair back from the hairline and pin it down securely with bobby pins.

Medium-length hair can be fastened in big pin curls. First comb your hair, then make two big parts, one from ear to ear, the other from center front to center nape. This gives you four sections. Take each section and make it into one or two big pin curls. Fasten them with bobby pins *pointed downward* so they won't snag on the wig when you put it on.

For really long hair, the best method is to wrap it around your head. Part your hair into four sections, parting from ear to ear and from center front to center back, holding each section separate with bobby pins. Now, starting with the right front section, wrap it into the left front section and around to the back, combing it as you go and securing with pins. As you comb and pin, pick up the right back section, then the left, and keep winding the hair until the whole thing is wrapped around your head like a smooth turban. Hold everything with bobby pins pointed *down.*

Now pull the wig on over your head like a swim cap. Be sure it's positioned properly, with the ear flaps directly opposite each other. Place it a little too far forward on your forehead. Then hold it at the hairline with one hand, and pull down at the nape with the other until the hairline is at the right place and looks like your own.

If you are going to use your own hair in the front pull it out with a rattail comb. Back-comb it lightly and gently mix it with the hair of the wig.

If the wig doesn't feel absolutely secure—which it should—a few big hairpins will give you extra security.

To take off a wig, take hold of it just in front of the ears and lift it straight up. Never pull it off by grabbing it by the hair.

Hairpieces

Hairpieces had a great period of popularity a few years ago. Everyone, it seemed, was wearing a fall. Or if she wasn't wearing it, she surely had one at home in her closet. Little curly pieces and pin-on chignons were almost as much in evidence. Now many people seem to think that hairpieces are finished. That isn't true. They're just not used as obviously as they were for a while when women wore two and three of them and styles were very elaborate and big.

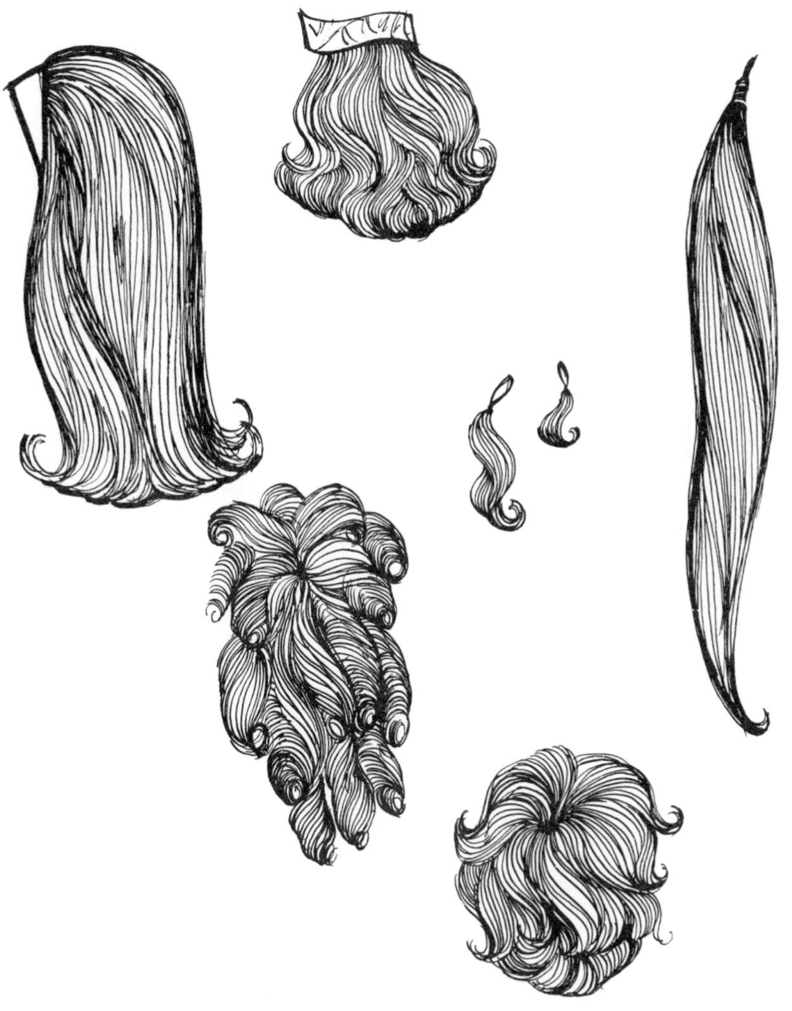

But they are still terribly useful. We use them all the time. Every model I know has a complete range of them, and uses them. I've done pages and pages of fashion pictures recently and I used hairpieces to get "instant" hairdos. I have dozens of clients who have invested thousands of dollars in them. They still use them, but they use them differently.

That's the point I want to make. Hairpieces are certainly not finished. I object to this age of "instant obsolescence" when things are momentarily "in" and then "out." Why toss away aids that free you from slavery to a hairdresser or to your hair, and give you the ability to look good easily and quickly and in all kinds of weather? Hairpieces are still great fashion accessories. All you must do is realize that the look of heads is different from what it was five years ago—it has become smaller. So you don't use a great big bulky hairpiece and make a great big head out of it. You use it to provide hair where you need it. And you use it in a more natural way, incorporated into your own hair, an integral part of it.

Hairpieces will give you more length, if that's what you want, or they will give you more bulk. They can be fillers for hair that is fine or thin or bodiless, or hair that doesn't stay in a set for more than a day. Once you get the hang of it, using a hairpiece is a tremendous convenience—you whip all your own hair up, stick a fall on and out you go. Or you mix it in with your own hair and look luxurious and real.

I am not a believer in using each hairpiece seven different ways, as advertised. Hairpieces are usually purchased by people who can't do anything much with their own hair, anyway, so how can these people be expected suddenly to become hairdressers? I think you should learn how to give yourself one terrific look with a hairpiece, something you can understand and cope with easily, and stick with it. If you want a different look, why not buy a different hairpiece? They're very inexpensive today. The idea of seven different looks from one hairpiece is, to my mind, a big sales pitch. Most people are not adept enough or interested enough for that. And they don't even want to look all those ways. They just want to look pretty.

The important thing to remember, as far as I'm concerned, is to know how to use each hairpiece to its best advantage. One way. If you can learn one good basic thing to do with your hairpiece a second idea will soon occur to you anyway.

The second important thing is that this false hair should look like your own hair, it should be a part of your head, not an attachment.

GETTING A GOOD MATCH: With the improvement in fibers and in manufacture, it is possible to get a hairpiece that blends into your own hair. The sheen must be the same. Many of the early synthetic pieces were much too shiny and, in the light, didn't integrate well. Today they're much better. And real hair, of course, doesn't usually have that problem.

The hair must be well matched in color. If it isn't don't buy it. There are so many colors, and more every day, that you can surely find one that goes with yours.

If you tint your hair you do have more of a problem because it is never the same color from week to week as it oxidizes. The best thing to do is to have the hairpiece matched in between colorings, perhaps two weeks after a bleaching or a tinting job so you will get a median shade.

Everyone's hair is lighter on the top and darkens as it gets nearer the roots. The hair that shows, the top layers, may be at least one shade and perhaps three or four shades lighter than the bottom layers. A hairpiece should be matched to the top.

Actually, I think that fake hair is going to improve all hair coloring. Manufacturers are taking such trouble to produce real hair colors for their wigs and hairpieces that they often look more real than the tints used on people's own hair—which are often pretty terrible. In fact, I think the colors of 90 per cent of the people who color their own hair look fake. Unfortunately, people have become used to the unreal colors and think they're better. I often look at a woman's hair and think it's a wig when it isn't. It's just some nasty coloring job.

To make a hairpiece match your own hair and look real, remember that you cannot attach a clean, wavy piece to dirty straight hair and have it look right. To mix successfully, it should be the same.

Falls

A fall is like half a wig. It covers half, or even three quarters or seven eighths of your head. Often with a fall you are showing only the front hairline of your own hair. You choose a fall according to how much you want to cover. It's really a hank of hair that you attach somewhere from just behind the hairline to the crown of your head, allowing the hair to fall to the back. It's perfect for people with short hair who want to have long hair temporarily, for hair that's not set but just brushed back and basically covered by the fall. The length can vary from about five inches to maybe thirty-six inches, all depending on what you want.

While a fall is usually used to get some length to the hair, it can be helpful as a filler for women who haven't got very heavy hair.

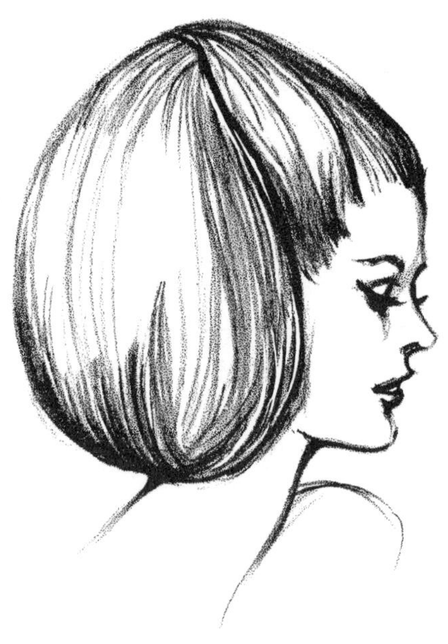

Brush your own front hair forward and attach the fall wherever you want the bulk to begin—usually at the back of the crown. Brush your own hair over it, teasing just a little.

Falls can be worn straight, curled (if they're real hair or one of the new curlable synthetics), waved, or braided or coiled or looped or made into pigtails. You can make them into little tiny braids or Shirley Temple curls. But do you really want to? I'd suggest having the fancy work done by an expert, especially if your fall is an expensive one, and that you save the elaborate arrangements only for special party occasions. It's best, I feel, to leave your fall alone and buy separate little braids, if you want them, or Shirley Temple curls, or whatever, rather than torment your fall.

Never tease a fall. And never permanent one. You can have anything done to a real-hair fall, even permanenting or bleaching or tinting, but take it to a good hairdresser and let him do the job.

If your fall is able to be set and you want some curl or wave in it, pin it to a wig block, dampen the ends and roll up on rollers. Dry it under a warm dryer. Then brush out gently.

When you buy a fall, you must choose the kind of base you want. Some bases only sit on top of your head, others cover the whole crown, and others are domed to give height. The shape could be round or triangular or oblong. Whatever the configuration, it must fit your head well.

Some of the bases are handmade. These, called ventilated, are usually thin, light and flexible and have much less bulk than machine-made caps. They're also more expensive and you will find them on real-hair falls and the better synthetic ones. The machine-made bases, called wefted, have a heavier base, both in bulk and weight, and consequently produce bigger bulk at the top of the head. That is what some people want because they produce instant height.

To use a fall and look like today, not 1965, think of placing it much farther back on your head than you did then. This allows your own hair to be sleeked back enough to see your natural head shape. The extra hair does not create excessive height or width and tends to look much more real, giving a better proportion. This doesn't mean that anyone should look like a pinhead either. Many people are hung up by the idea that they need height. This may be true with their own shorter hair but remember that when you add length and softness around the chin and neck area you don't need the bulk on top.

Wiglets

These are smaller and shorter hairpieces and, while falls have swing and movement, wiglets are usually wavy or curly and on a flat base. They are lightweight and easy to handle. In different sizes, they are used as fillers providing bulk and body or height

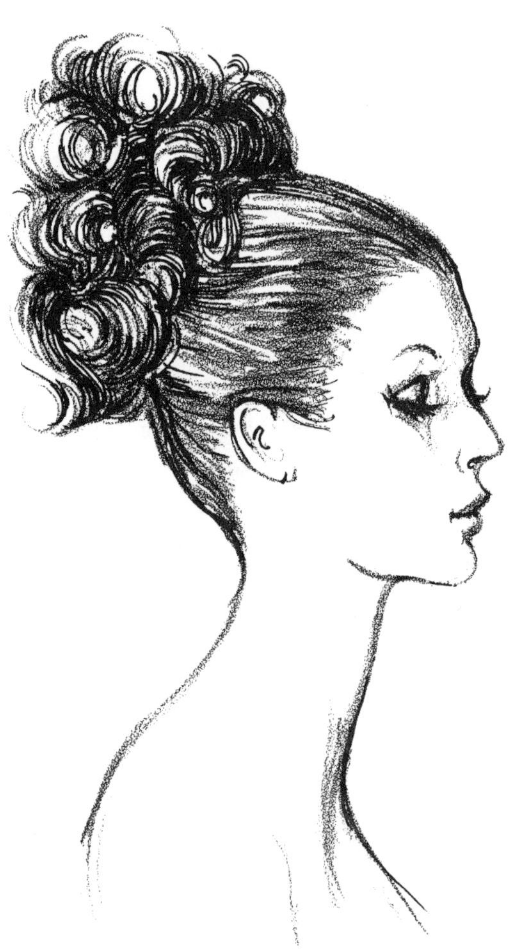

wherever you need it. Or they are used as decoration, as in an evening hairdo with clusters of curls. They are designed to be literally incorporated into your own hair, which is mixed in with it. You might even wear two at a time if you want more fantasy.

Cascades

A larger wiglet with a long rectangular base, for people who want more coverage from top to bottom or side to side.

Switches

Long hanks of hair which can be worn plain, or braided or twisted into a chignon of any configuration.

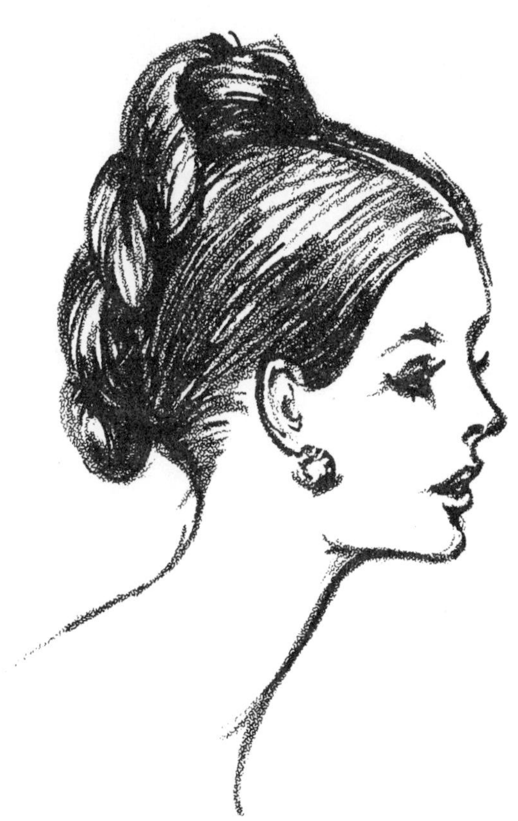

Cluster Curls

Three or four curls—or sometimes even just one—on a hairpin base, to be stuck in your hairdo wherever you need them. Store them wound around a roller.

Ponytail Clip-Ons

In varying lengths, these can simply be snapped on to the back of your head.

Plus other small hairpieces such as bangs and coils and ringlets.

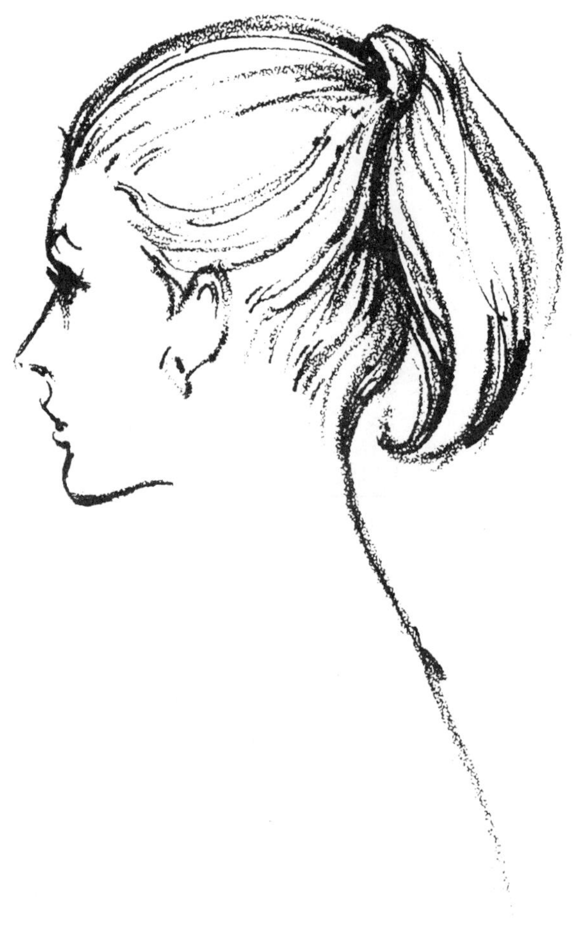

Attaching Hairpieces

One of the best ways I know to attach a fall or a smaller hairpiece is to make two or three flat pin curls, holding them with crisscrossed bobby pins. If the piece has a comb in it—and most do—slide the comb under the bobby pins and put a few long hairpins right through the mesh of the backing and into the pin curls. Be careful not to tear the base by forcing the hairpins through it.

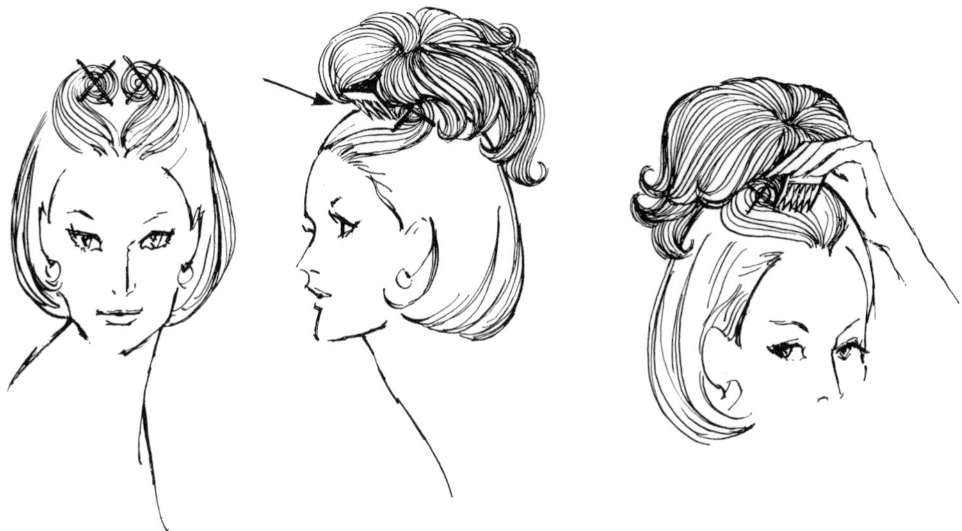

If the piece does not have a comb hold it in place with two or three bobby pins around the edges.

If there is a discernible demarcation where the new hair begins, as there is with a fall, cover it with a hairband or a ribbon or a strip of the hair twisted around. Or blend the front of your own hair in with the fall. If you're going to do this take a section of your own front hair, perhaps two inches wide, and comb it forward before you make the pin curls. Hold it with a clip. Then make the pin curls behind this section. Attach the fall. Now brush the front hair back over the fall. Usually you must tease it slightly to get it to stay together and in the right place.

A wiglet must be disguised by teasing your own surrounding hair and lightly brushing into the edges of the hairpiece.

To wear a chignon, comb your own hair into the shape you want—usually its pulled back with bobby pins or into a flat French twist. Spray it now so you won't have to spray the hairpiece. Now attach the chignon with long hairpins all around the edges.

The ponytails are merely snapped on to your own hair in back.

The hairpins of the cluster curls are stuck into your own hair and held with a bobby pin.

To attach a long braid, there are several methods. One is to pull your own hair back and into a French twist. Then pin the hairpiece at the top of the twist, adding a few hairpins down the braid and into the twist for security.

Another: Gather your own hair into a little knot high on the back of your head. Attach the braid in front of this knot with hairpins, pinning a little way down the head to keep it in place.

Wig Accessories

For an acrylic wig, which you bought because it's a convenience and doesn't require an enormous investment, you don't really need anything more than some wig shampoo and a good wig brush. The wig will probably come in a box. Just store it, stuffed with tissue paper, sitting upside down in the box. Or hang it up on something—like a doorknob. As a matter of fact, you don't even need a special shampoo or a special brush—though a wire brush does seem to work best.

Beyond this, there are many other accessories you can get if you feel the need, and if you have a place to keep them. There are wig blocks, and carrying cases, and wig liners, and wig lift combs and wig chin straps. My feeling is: Do what's easiest for you and don't let yourself be talked into a lot of stuff that will probably just lie about in your room or further stuff your drawers or closets.

Chapter 10

CLASSIC HAIR STYLES

There are several hair styles which I call classic because they have remained—or will remain—popular for many years. They are classic because they last—with variations, of course; and they last because they look good on a lot of people, they are comfortable and easy to maintain.

Unfortunately many good hair styles don't make it as classics because they become *too* popular too fast. Nothing kills a fashion more thoroughly than that. If you see every other woman wearing the same hairdo, especially if it is a very definite or exaggerated style, the eye quickly tires of it. It begins to look as though it's a hairdo made by a cookie cutter. That's what happened with the Shag cut—it came in with a holler and went right out because it soon looked like a shag machine was turning it out. Besides, most of the Shags were so badly done. You'd see one beautiful Shag cut and three thousand terrible ones.

The same happened with the Gibson girl upsweep. It was lovely when it first appeared. Then it became a fad, usually overdone and too exaggerated, or messy and more like something you'd wear in the shower than a hairdo. It was done in by its popularity.

The real classics, I've found, are the simple hair styles, such as these:

The French Twist

This is a way for women with long hair to have a neat and tidy head with distinct definition. It gives an uncluttered kind of look and a quiet elegance, showing off a beautiful head shape or a lovely long neck to full advantage. It has been with us for many years and has had repeated popular revivals. Because it's so simple, it's not good for someone who needs "help" from her hair, who looks best with softness around the face. And it requires a careful and artful makeup job for the same reason. Your face, especially your eyes, must be emphasized.

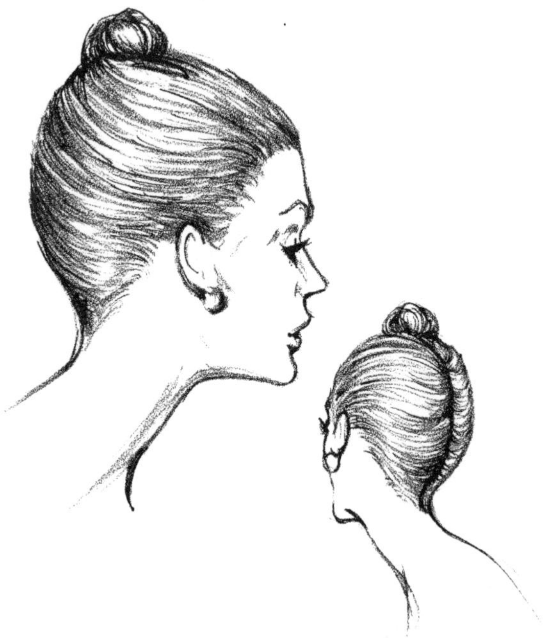

A French twist, I feel, looks best on darker shades of hair, and it has to be very, very neat. The finished shape is small, so this is not a style for those who feel they must have height or width or bulk.

Nor is it for anyone with a badly shaped head—it really does follow the contours of the head.

Brush all your hair back and upward to the back of the crown. Catch it together in your hand. Then twist that hair in either direction, and keep twisting until the hair is all tightened. As you do this, pull it up. Now what you have is a long twist up the back of your head, looking rather like a fold. Secure this with bobby pins or hairpins all along the edge. Then wrap the ends of the hair into a flat chignon, tucking them in so it looks like a continuous twist. Or if the ends are curly, you can leave a few soft curls up top—but never anything big or elaborate. The charm of the French twist is its utter simplicity.

The Chignon

This is the hairdo of the ballerina, probably the most classic style of all. It's as personal a hairdo as it's possible to achieve and I think it is extremely feminine. I know many beautiful women who wear this style, no matter whether their friends appear in bouffants, serf cuts, tendrils or shags. It is often very good on someone who is

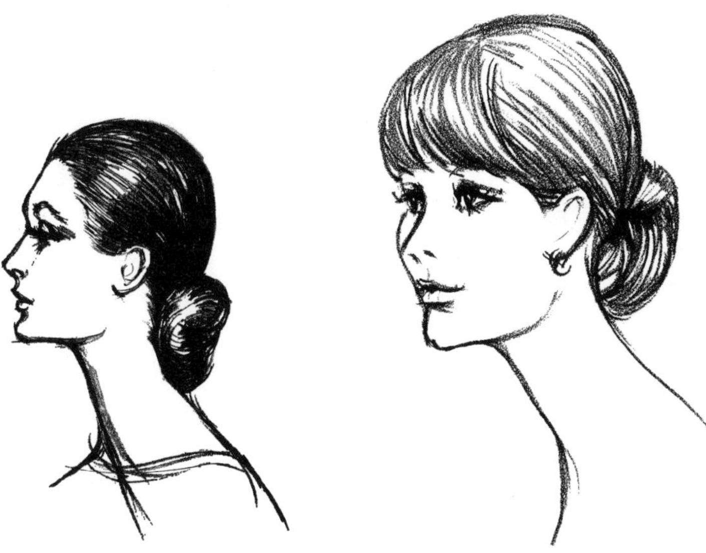

pretty but just doesn't have the extra flair that makes her a beauty. It often works well on a woman with a prominent nose, making what might be considered a bad feature into one that's interesting and attractive. It does need delineation of the eyes and perhaps a brighter mouth than you are used to.

This hair style does not require a set unless you'd like more body in your hair. Pull the hair back and catch it in a covered elastic at the nape. Your hair shouldn't be terribly long because the chignon looks best if it's not too large. If the hair is at least six inches below the elastic, twist it around in one piece until it turns itself into its own "bun." Pin in place, tucking the ends underneath. Experiment with various shapes.

If your hair isn't long enough to do this, if you have only a few

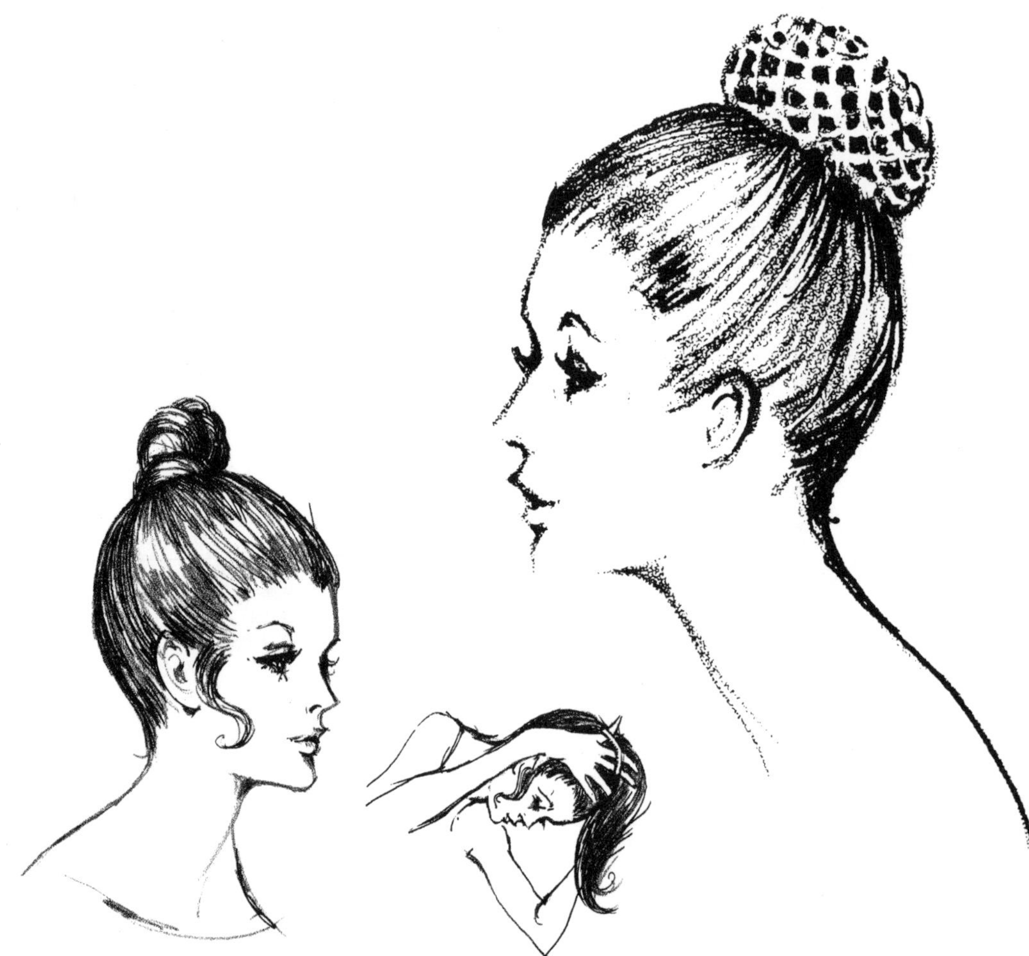

inches left over, take it and turn it under into a tight little roll, making it really solid. Pin in place. Then wrap a fake switch around the outside, perhaps braiding it first.

The chignon or bun can be placed anywhere on your head if your hair is long enough, letting little ends fall into tendrils. Try pulling it up on top of your head or to the back.

Ponytail

This has become a classic too, because it's a way of containing the hair, of getting it out of the way. It's expedient and can be beautiful if you pay close attention to your makeup.

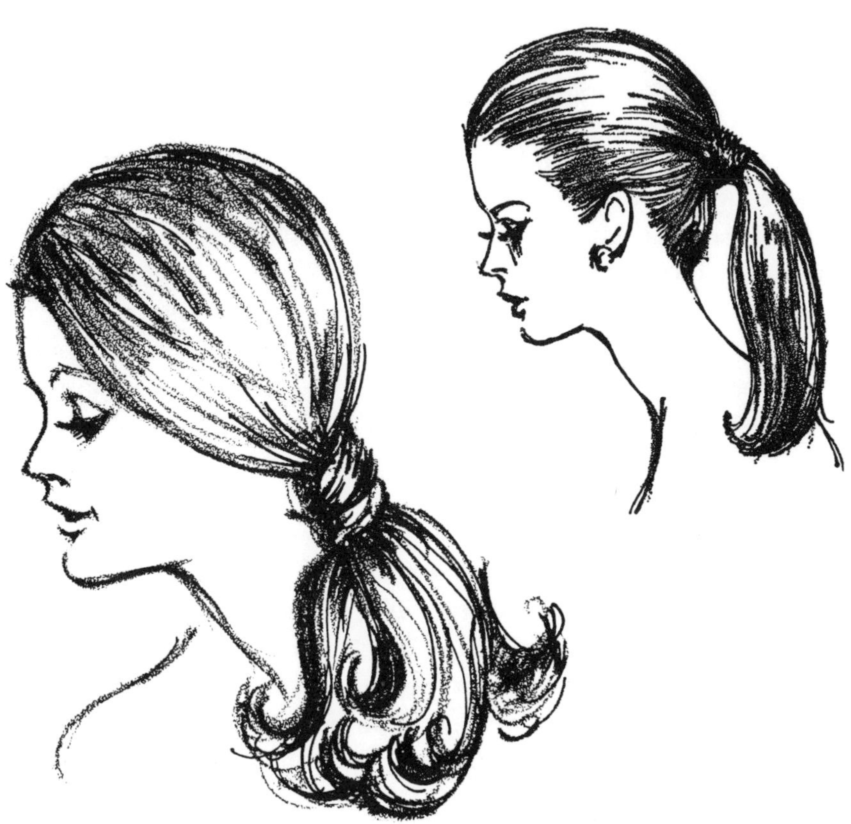

The tail can be worn high on your head, raised a bit above the nape, or very low in a George Washington. Catch the hair in a covered elastic, then cover that with a scarf, a ribbon or other ornament. Sometimes it's pretty if you cover the entire "tail" with a looped scarf.

While some women can wear their hair pulled straight back and flat to the head, most feel the need for a bit of volume. If you do, set the crown straight back or slightly angled to the side on large rollers. If necessary, tease the crown a little. For curly ends, roll these up too. Make tendrils out of little pieces that won't stay in the elastic by putting them up in pin curls.

Always remember, though, that the more you do to "fancy up" a ponytail hairdo, the further away you get from what you probably really wanted to begin with: a simple, casual look.

Very Long, Swinging Hair

This is almost universal for young girls now. It is the uniform of today. I happen to think that long hair is great—if it's pretty. That means it can't be tangled, unkempt, a thousand lengths, three or four colors, dirty or even slightly soiled. It will look wonderful if it's well shaped and doesn't appear to have been touched by a hairdresser. It should never look anything like a hairdo, just as the makeup that goes with it shouldn't look like makeup.

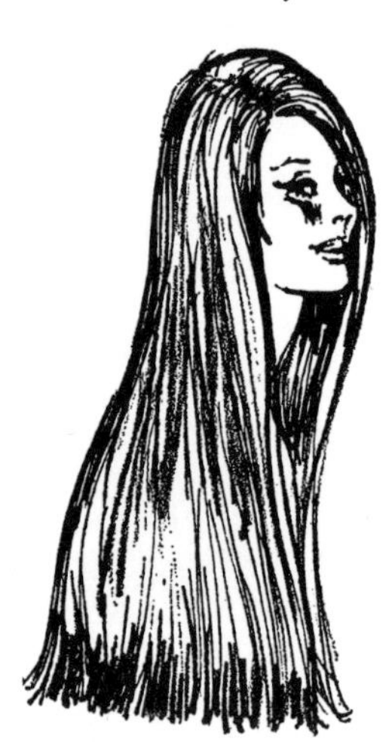

Not everyone can manage long hair. You have to consider your body proportions. If you are a little tiny girl with no neck and if you're a little heavier than you ought to be, you will look awful, because the longer the hair the shorter your proportions seem. If your only problem is a short neck, then you must do something to raise your neck

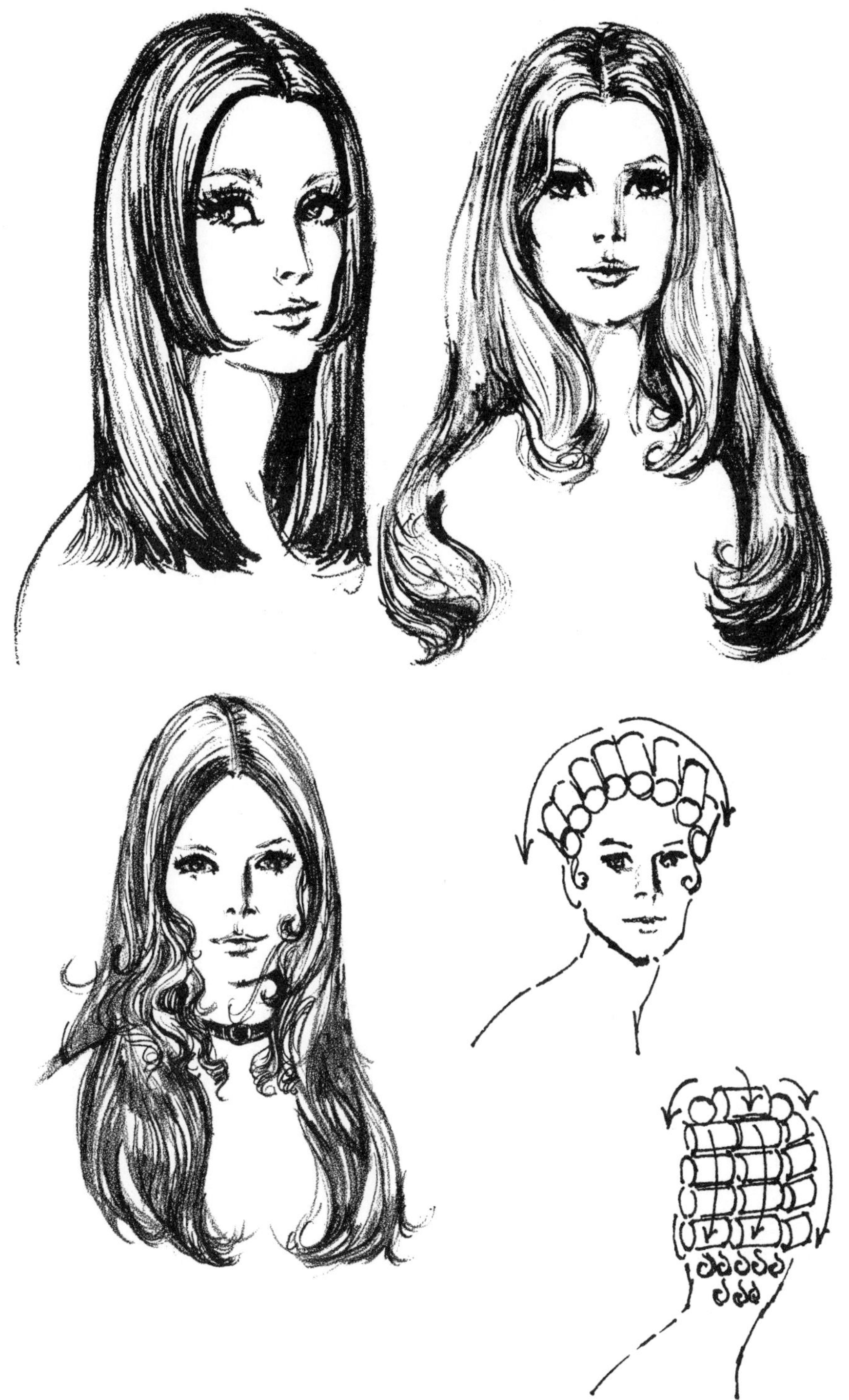

from your shoulders, and so you should pull your hair up and away from the neck in some manner.

There is a myth that hair grows more quickly if you don't cut it. That's not true. Your hair needs to be cut, perhaps only a quarter of an inch, about every six weeks. Hair always tends to break or split at the ends. Besides, it doesn't grow evenly.

Long hair should swing or move like a tassel or a piece of fabric. For this it needs a blunt even cut, slightly shorter in back, with no layering at all.

Just plain long hair isn't flattering to everyone. Sometimes, too, it looks a little messy. A good solution to the problem is to have two-level hair. This is where the hair is long and swinging, cut perhaps to the shoulders or below, with some hair cut a shorter length at cheek or chin length. What this accomplishes is the look of long hair but with a certain softness and flattery around the face. Besides, it solves the problem of hair that is always falling in your face. For someone who wants to pull her hair back but looks stark that way, it's ideal.

You have to be sensible about how short and how deep the shorter length should be. There are three things to take into consideration. One is, of course, the shape of hair you want. Another is the texture of your hair. And the third is that you must leave the shorter level long enough to push behind your ear if a cleaner, smoother look is what you want sometimes.

For instance, let's take the example of someone who has a fairly wide jaw. In order to cut into that width, the shorter hair should hit just a speck below the jawbones. If her hair is fine in texture she would need more hair in the shorter length than someone with coarser hair; in other words, there should be a wider section cut short. Otherwise it will look too wispy and won't be manageable.

This is how a lot of fashion models wear their hair today, as it helps create different looks easily.

Now, how should you treat this second level of hair? You can leave it straight, of course. You can curl it slightly. Or you can curl it tightly and get tendrils out of it. It can be rolled on rollers with the rest of the hair, or done with big flat pin curls. Or it may be treated as a heavy *guiche* and allowed to dry almost straight, perhaps held in place with tape. I think the prettiest and youngest way is to have it flow with the rest of the hair and not become a separate element.

Again, I believe in a very blunt, even haircut and, most certainly, a good blunt cut on the shorter level so that it lies on the face and has a luxurious quality about it.

Short Curly Hair

This is a classic because of the ease in caring for it and because it can look good whether you're fourteen or seventy.

Usually hair is layered in even lengths all over the head, about two to four inches long. This doesn't mean the finished length is all the same; it means each hair whether on the crown or at the

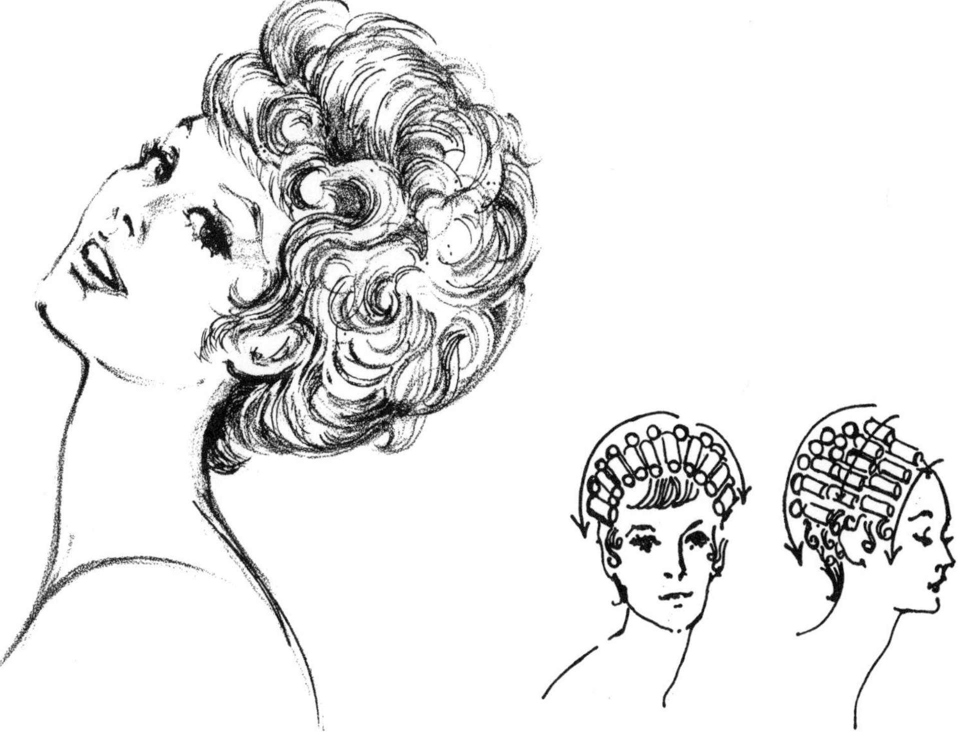

sides or top is the same length from root to end. The back, however, could be closely cropped or it could be a little longer to give a softer look.

Obviously, a person whose hair is naturally curly will find this hair style the easiest to live with. If your hair isn't curly you'll probably need a permanent wave, if you don't want to be constantly setting it. If you do set it, use rather small rollers or tight pin curls. It is best if it doesn't look set or arranged, so when you comb it out after a setting, use your fingers to pull out little pieces here and there.

Short Straight, or Fairly Straight, Hair

Here is another classic, with endless variations. We've been through many versions of it for the last twenty years, starting with the cap cut, then the gamin, right up to the short crop popularized

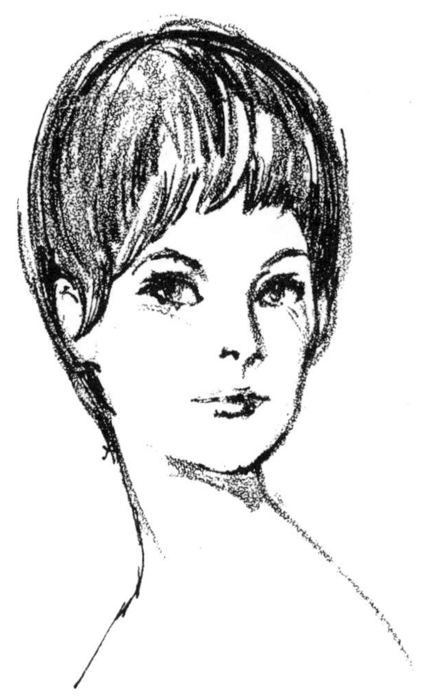

by Mia Farrow. This is probably the easiest in the world to care for, except that it must be cut on a very regular basis, every three to four weeks. It's a wash-and-wear style, though you may want to add a couple of rollers or pin curls occasionally just for a change of look.

The ideal short straight hair doesn't need setting at all, but can be combed into place. Comb some setting lotion through your hair after you've towel-dried it, just for body to hold it in line while it dries completely. Or you can blow it dry.

Short hair has to have a superb cut because you can't camouflage a bad shape. If the cut is bad, no amount of fussing will do much good. This style must be very simple and you can't expect always to get the most flattering one for you. But remember the convenience. And certainly not everyone can wear a short, close style. A girl with a large head and a round face would look terrible this way. So would a very tall large girl because her head would look too small in proportion to her body. And, in general, it's more a style for the young who don't need a very soft look around the face.

All-One-Length Hair

Hair that is all one length at the bottom edges has become an American classic. For the past ten years, the younger woman has preferred longer hair and she still does. If her hair is all one length this longer hair is easier to manage. Generally all she needs to do is shampoo it, dry it and brush it.

This kind of hair has made people very hair conscious and has probably been the single most important factor in the new direction of hairdressing. It will last for a long time, while other, more extreme or more difficult, hair styles will pass. All-one-length hair is the kind of style that shows off really beautiful hair to its best advantage. It moves nicely on the head, it swings. It is so simple, so graphic, so dependent on the haircut and the woman's own ability to care for it that it makes its owner conscious of the texture, the body or lack of body, the curl, the wave, the health, the condition.

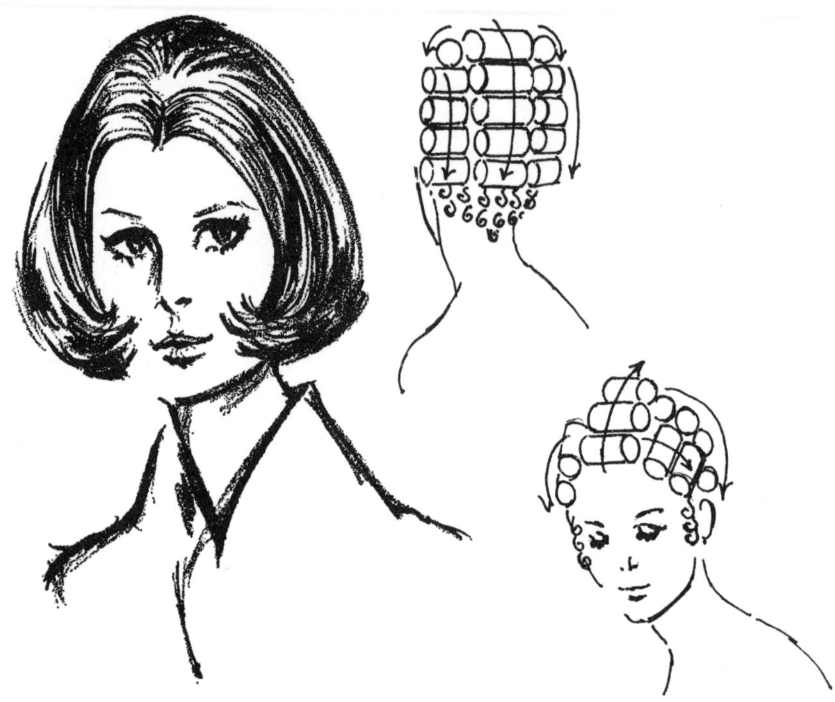

It is very blunt-cut hair, with the finished length anywhere from just below the ears to the shoulders. It's usually worn fairly straight, because anyone wearing this style is usually aiming for a very free "natural" look. But it can be set on big rollers all over the head as well as wrapped or blown dry.

It can be cut to hang evenly all around the head, but often it's given more exaggerated shape and line by making it shorter in the back, longer toward the front; or vice versa, longer in the back and shorter toward the front. The graduation in length may be hardly noticeable or greatly exaggerated.

The Afro

Many black women, and men too, have abandoned hair straighteners and wear their hair short and curly in what's called the Afro or the natural. And it can look beautiful. There is no one Afro

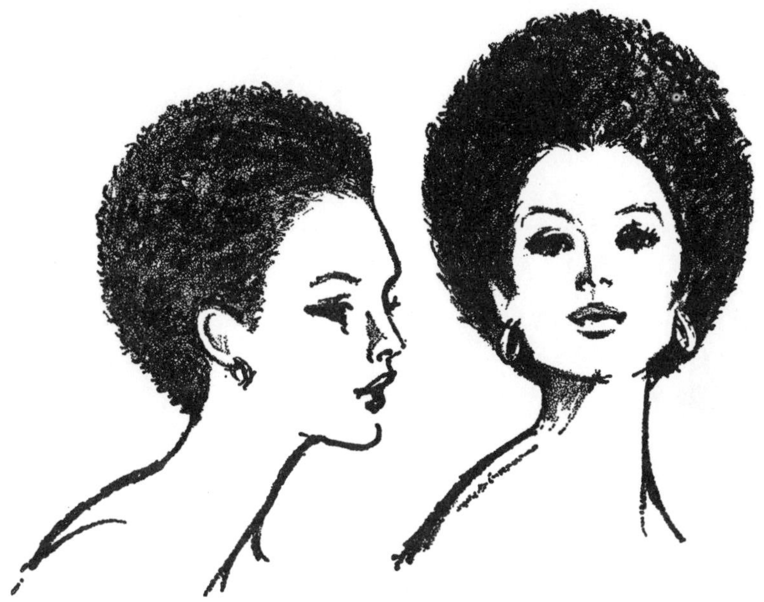

shape—the idea is to make the shape of your hair one which suits you—your personality and your face and your body proportions, perhaps even your mood of the moment. I include the Afro as a classic because it has become so widely worn and I think it will continue to be. While I understand that in the very beginning of its popularity it was a visual sign of freedom, now it has become a fashion. Consequently, we do see many forms of it as people try to make their hair into individual but flattering shapes.

Let me warn you, not every black girl can wear her hair this way to great advantage. This looks best on a slim, elegantly tall and well-proportioned woman because there's a regal quality about it. You can't be too wide or have a heavy neck and look good in all forms of it.

You must also consider whether your hair adapts to this style. Like Caucasian and Oriental hair, black people's hair is not all the same. It ranges from a distinct tight curl pattern to bone straight, from coarse to fine in texture.

The hairdo is strictly a cut. The hair is washed first, then brushed dry. Then it is clipped and sculpted with scissors. I like an

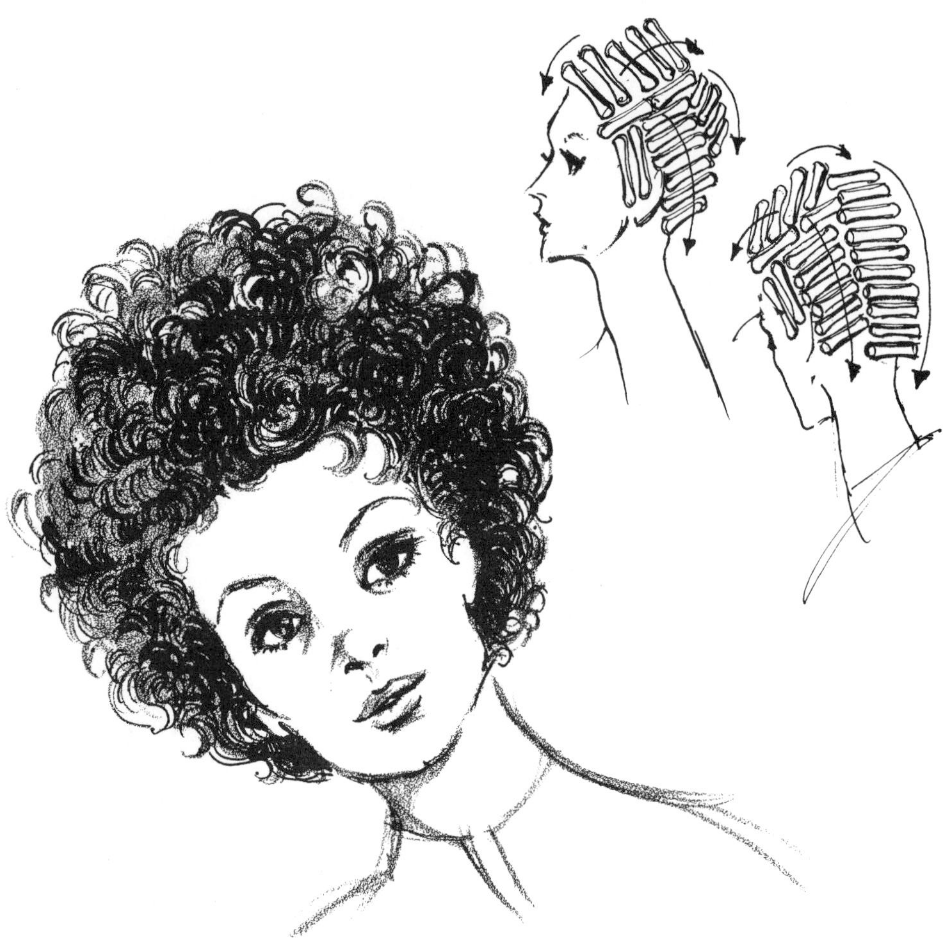

almost round quality rather like a spaceman's helmet, with the nape cut closer to give the head a delineation, rather than an allover halo look. But you can develop your own shape. Fiddle around with it, pat it and push it, pull little pieces out here and there, until it is right for you.

If your hair isn't curly enough to make a good Afro you can set it. Use permanent-wave rods to get a very strong wave. Then back-comb the hair thoroughly and make a shape out of it. Some people set this style by making tiny tight braids all over the head, then undoing them and pulling the hair into a shape.

Long-Short Hair

Hair that is short in front and on the sides and longer in the back can look many different ways. For example:

The Serf cut, which can be quite short or quite long. To get this look, your hair must be fairly long to start with, because the length at the nape must be at least four inches so that the hair behind your ears can be seen from the front. It is cut almost in a circle from the center of the crown. It's a blunt cut with just a touch of layering for bounce. The bangs, too, come from the center crown, giving a sense of luxury to the hair. When you comb it, it must be soft and fluffy with little bits of the hair going this way and that, so you don't look as if you're wearing a hat.

The Serf cut—if it's soft—makes the eyes big and marvelous.

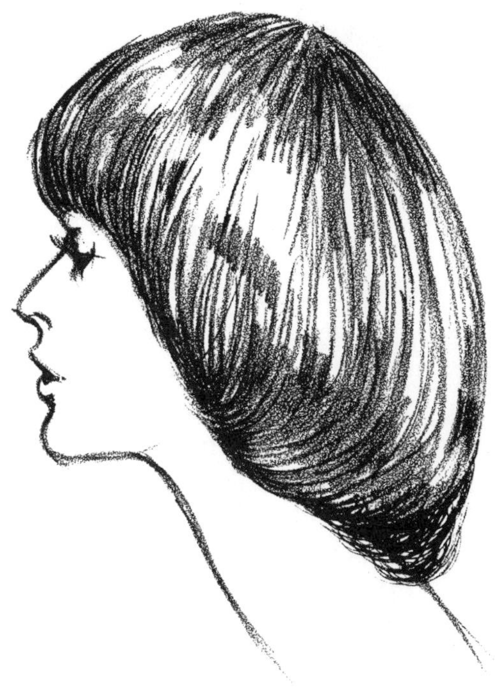

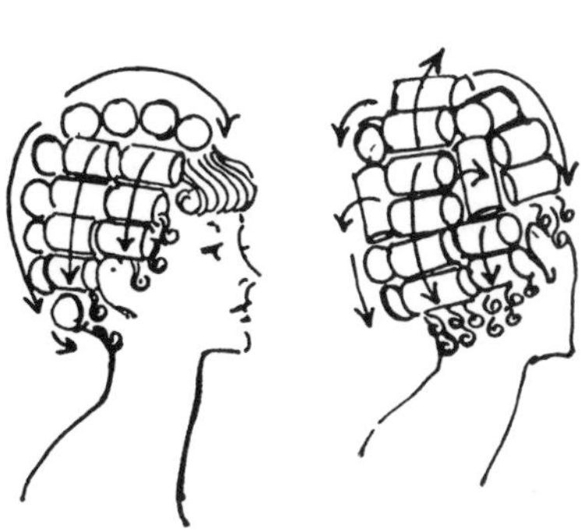

It's a good hairdo for camouflaging an unattractively low forehead because the bangs start so far back that one never knows where your forehead begins. And it's also a good style for fine hair. If your hair is dark, I think highlights right around the face will make it much prettier. I don't mean blond streaks but some shading just a little lighter than your own color.

This cut may need only to be washed often and blown dry. Be sure your hair is always very clean so it doesn't stick together and look heavy. If you need to set it use curlers that are one and a half to two inches in diameter, depending on the texture of your hair. Use a smaller roller if your hair is hard to curl. If your hair takes a set easily I suggest that some of the bangs be put over cotton instead of rollers so they won't jump up too much. The cotton will give a slight lift without actually curling them.

Brush the hair well, out from the center. Don't tease it, except perhaps a tiny bit at the crown if you need a little lift. Just let the hair fall freely around your face.

The Napoleonic, Empire, whatever you call it, is a long-short hair style that's on its way to becoming a classic because it looks so good on so many people. It's the newest approach to haircutting where the bottom length, or controlling length, can be anywhere from chin to shoulder and the rest of the hair is layered above that.

It can be worn smooth and fairly close to the head with exaggerated length around the entire hairline, giving a soft shagginess to the head. It can be worn nearly straight, or it can be curled very tightly. It can have height and be worn away from the face, or it can be combed into deep bangs. This is a very individual style, depending first on your own look and then on the texture of your hair. There are people whose hair can be cut this way and then simply blown dry. There are others who need more wave and curl and consequently need to set their hair. Sometimes this haircut is very exaggerated with the bottom layers very long and the top extremely short. Just keep in mind that this exaggeration is only for the very young.

More than any other hair style, this one is based on healthy

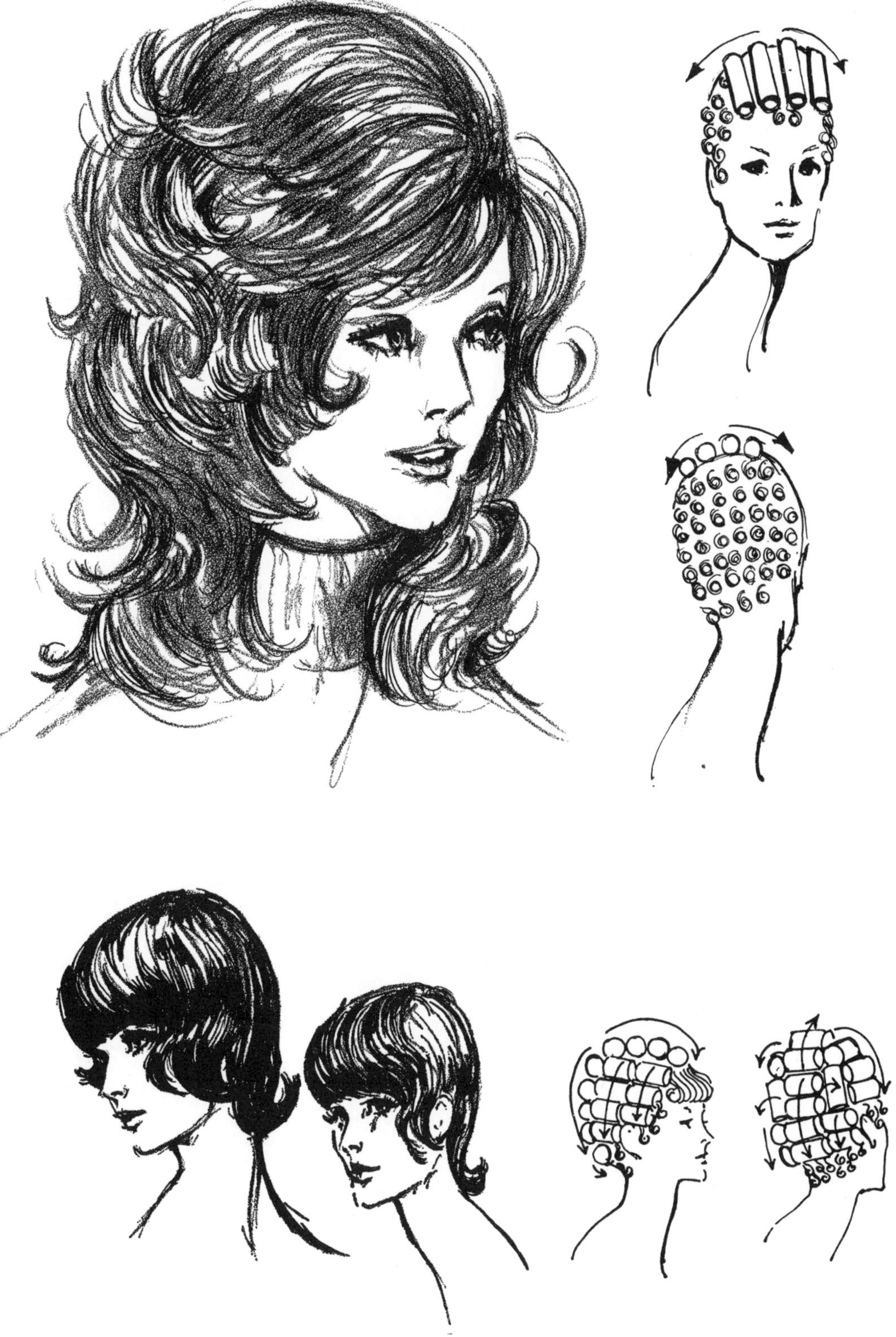

hair. I mean really shiny, clean, strong hair. It's not pretty otherwise. In fact, it won't work unless the hair is in great condition. But it can look great on very fine hair.

Most important, this style depends almost totally on a superb haircut, one that's painstakingly achieved. It's not something you can do at home with a pair of manicure scissors. It needs a professional haircut.

This long-short hair can look pretty awful if it isn't carefully layered, if the bottom lengths straggle down the neck while the others are much shorter. I am *not* talking about the Shag. You should hardly be able to tell the difference in lengths.

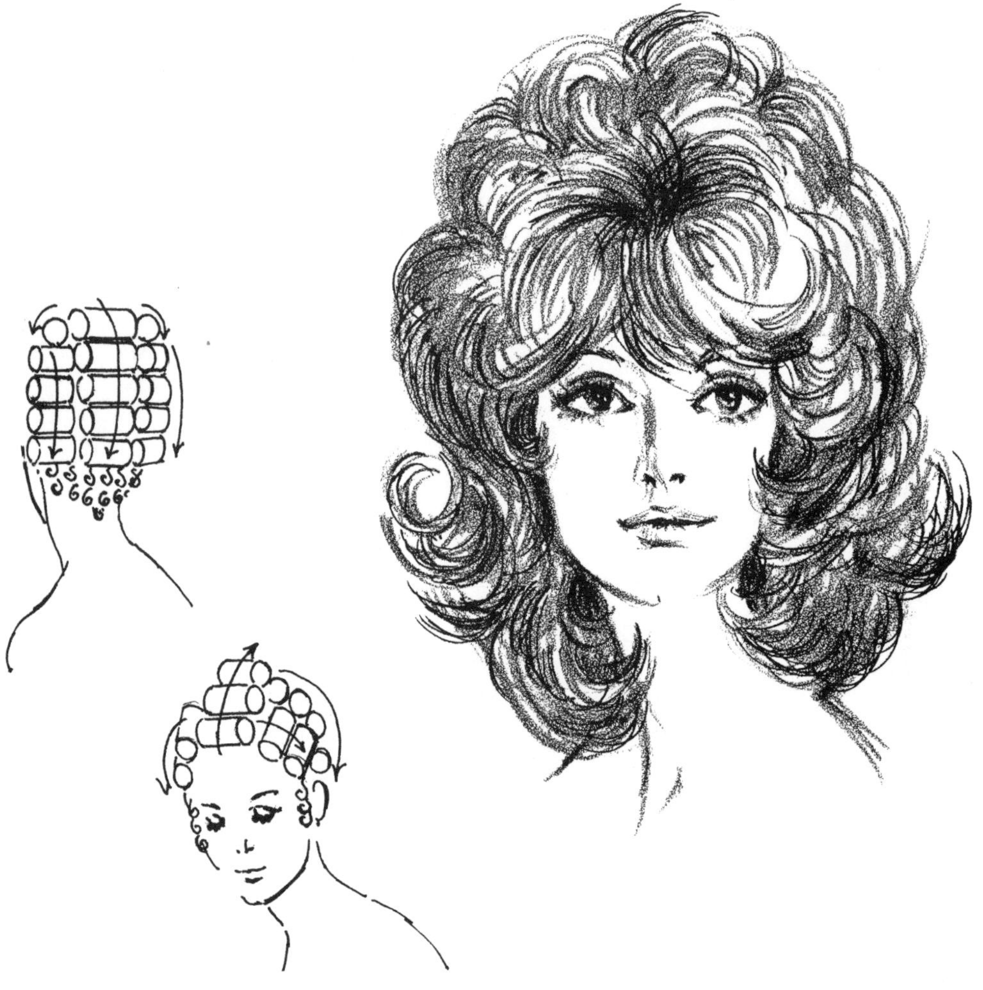

To set this hair—if you need to—you can go in almost any direction, setting the top on smaller rollers and switching to a larger size at the bottom. You can also set the hair with pin curls all over the head. It can be blown dry without any curling for a really straight look very close to the head. Or you can then put just a few heated rollers in any area where you might want lift or a bit of bend.

MY PORTFOLIO OF HAIR STYLES

Here's a collection of hair styles I've created, most of which have appeared in national magazines, some on the covers. As you can see, I feel that pretty hair isn't any one style or look. It can reflect a range of moods and a range of shapes. Always remember: There's not just one hairdo for you. Any style can be contemporary if it suits you, your life style and your own particular hair texture, so there's no need to try for the "latest" hairdo. To prove this, take a look at the photographs here. Some appeared as early as 1965, and others just this year. I chose them because they show a certain evolution that's occurred in hair fashion in the last ten years, and because they demonstrate that a good hair style is really timeless. And, finally, they can tell you better than words what I think is pretty hair.

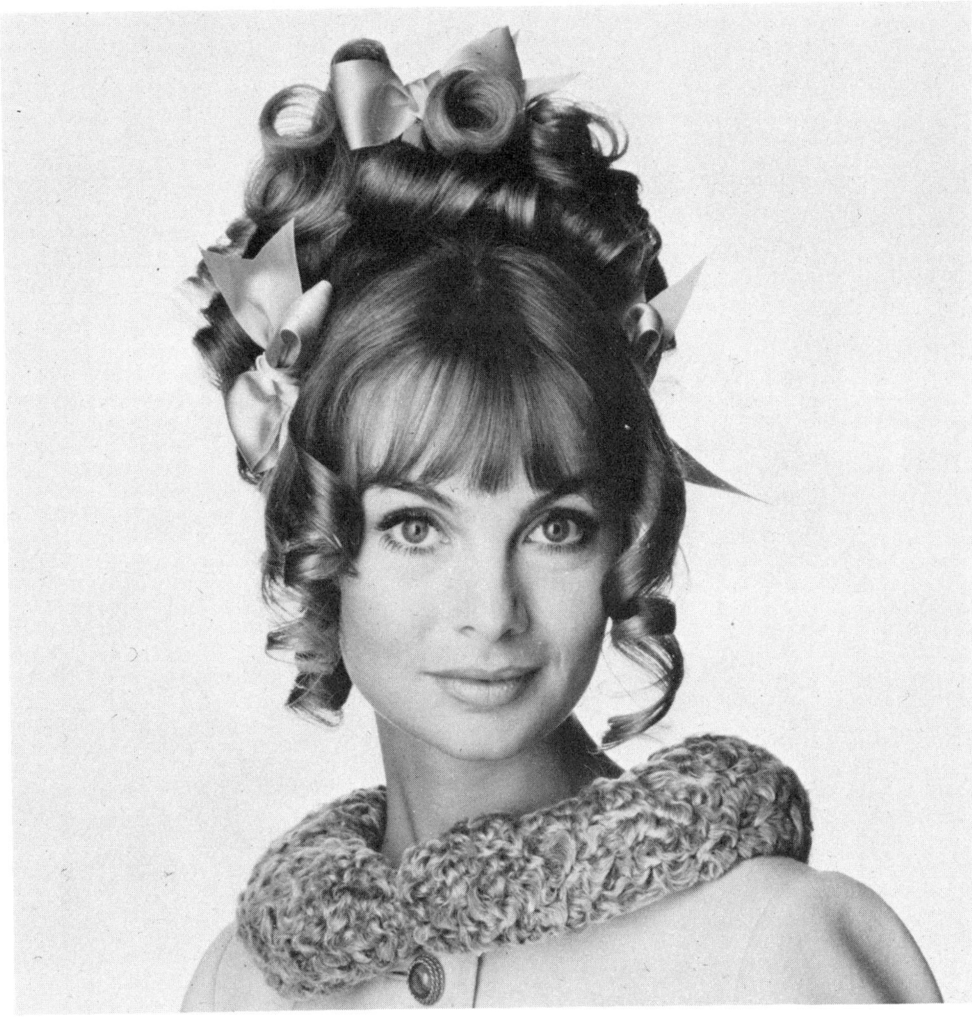

This was a *Vogue* cover on Jean Shrimpton. I think this hairdo has an ageless quality. It's the kind of hairdo so many women feel is pretty or feminine. Of course, it's for evening. From *Vogue*, © 1967 by The Condé Nast Publications, Inc. Photographer: David Bailey

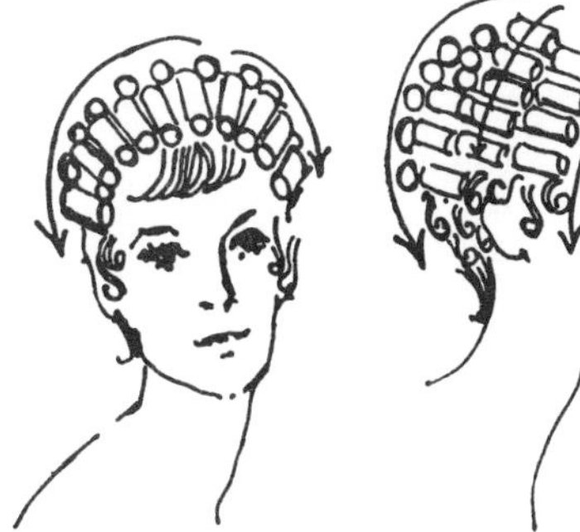

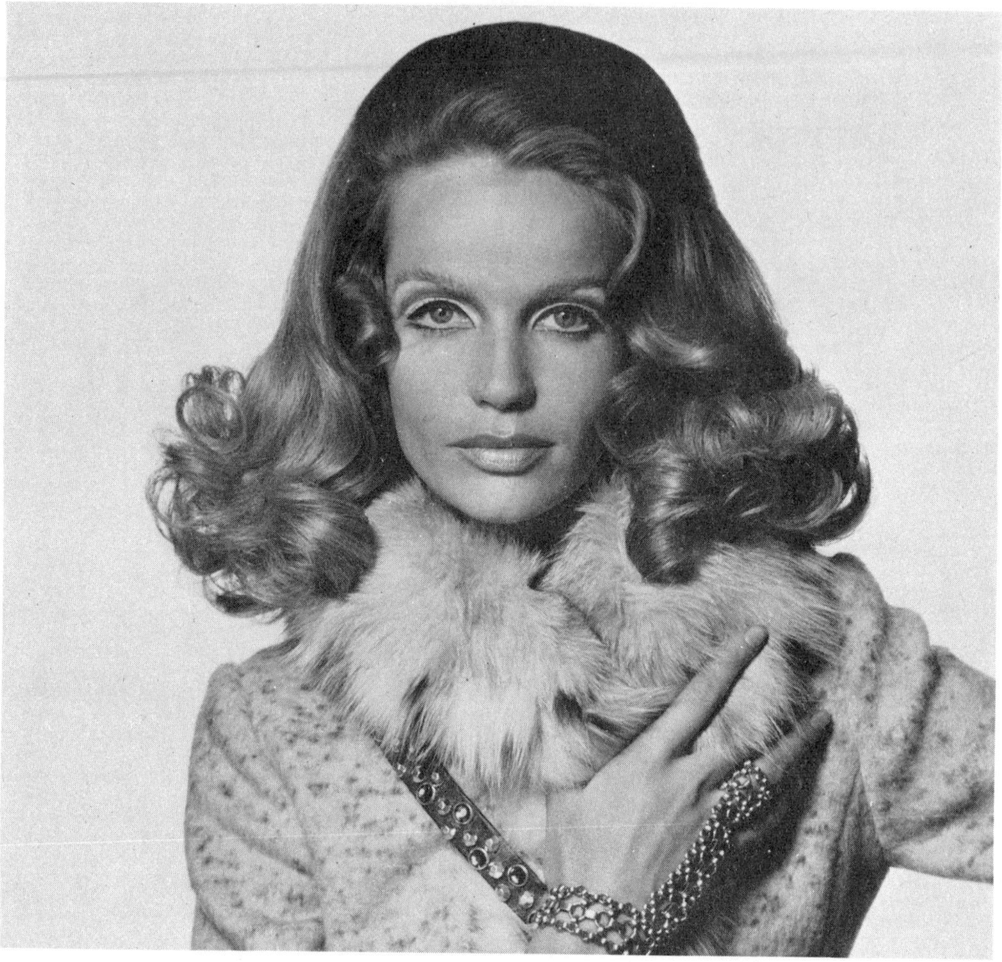

Another *Vogue* cover, this time on Verushka, one of my favorite models. I chose this as I think it represents classic soft, medium-length hair that almost any age can wear. I like the feeling of luxury. This would, of course, be hard to achieve with poor-quality or thin hair, but even then you could do it with the help of a fall. From *Vogue*, © 1968 by The Condé Nast Publications, Inc.

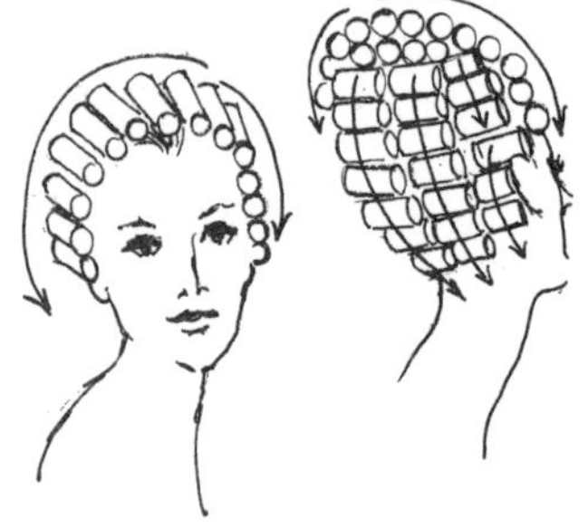

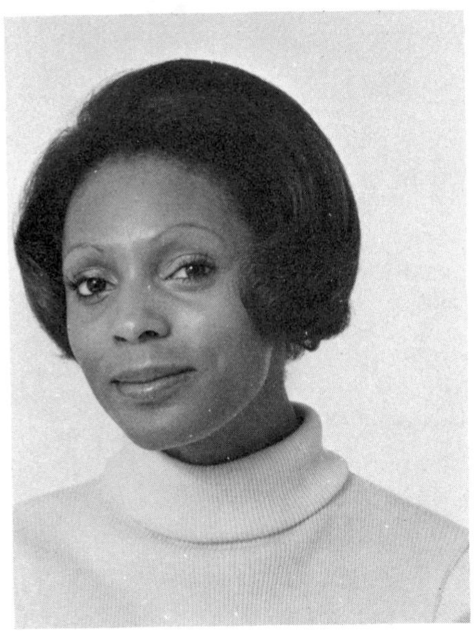

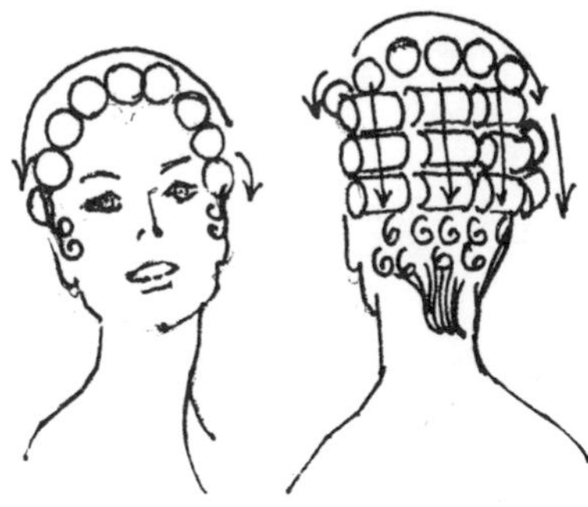

For very curly medium-length hair, this must be set on large rollers (1½ to 2″) to stretch out the curl, aided by a strong setting lotion. Usually this kind of hair doesn't have to be back-combed, but it can be if your hair doesn't hold together well. *Woman's Day,* June 1971. Photographer: William Connors

Here we've added a little wiglet at the nape for a more dressed-up look. It's always important to remember, when you're adding a hairpiece, that it must blend perfectly with your own hair so it won't look like an addition. *Woman's Day,* June 1971. Photographer: William Connors

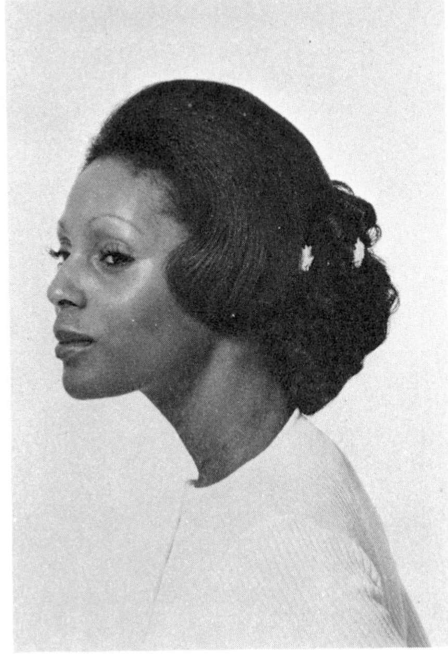

One of my favorite looks for the more mature woman who does not want to settle for a little cropped curly hairdo. This can be done with almost any texture of hair, but always remember: the finer the hair, the smaller the rollers. *McCall's Magazine*, March 1969. Photographer: Art Kane

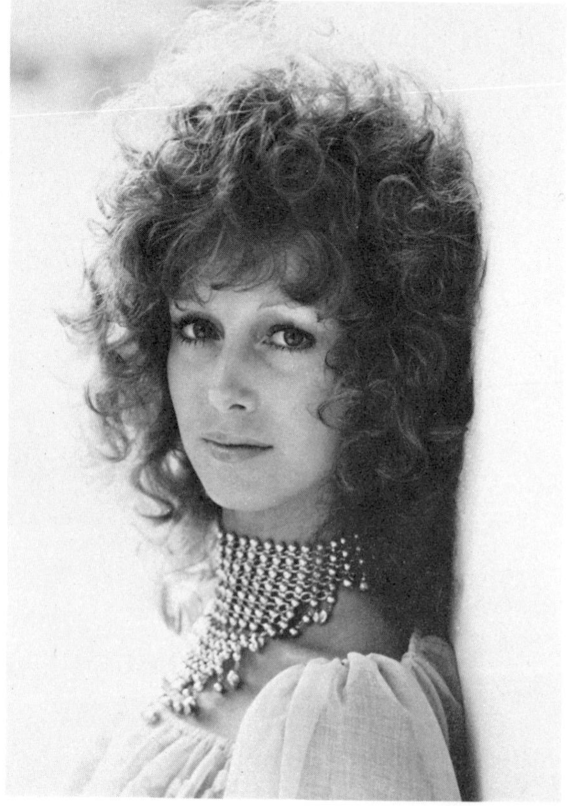

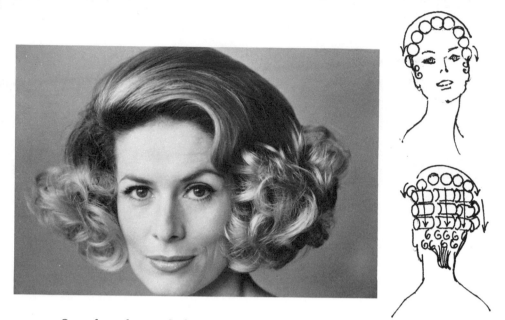

A hairdo for a girl who has wispy hair that never stays straight but also has no body. It's set on permanent-wave rods, then brushed through and arranged with the fingers. *Woman's Day*, June 1971. Photographer: William Connors

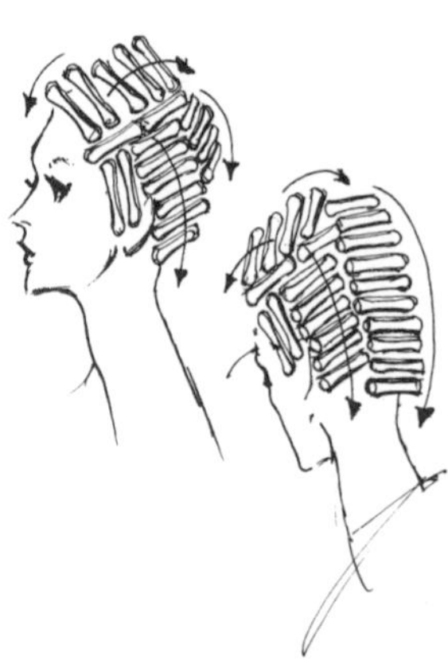

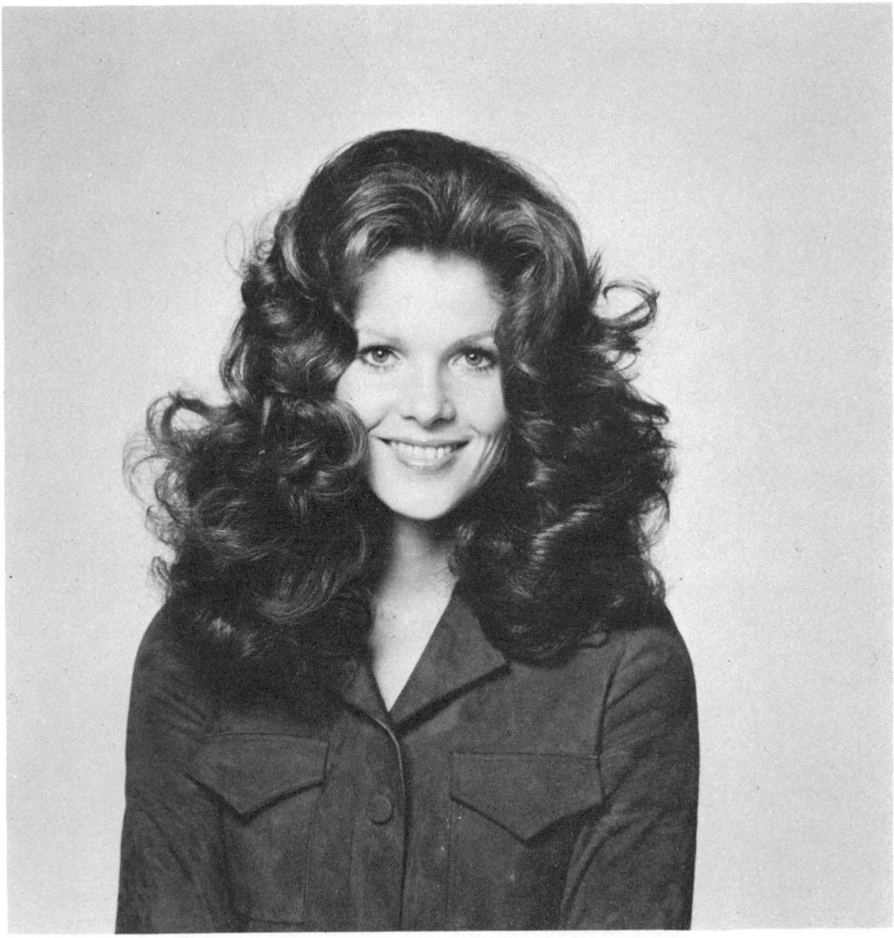

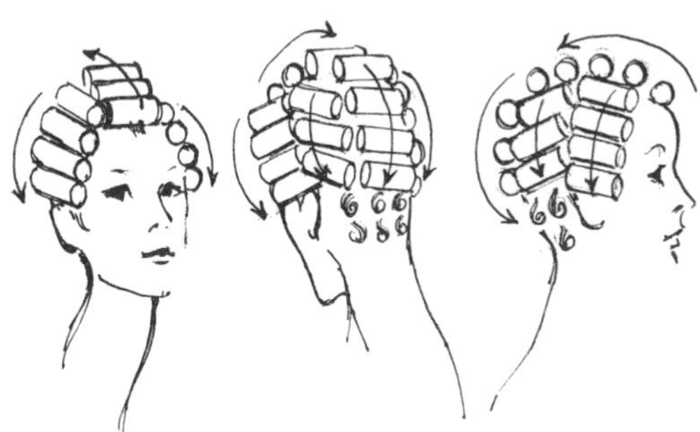

Basically a familiar hair style, this is the way many women have worn their hair for quite a few years. But it's done on rollers today instead of pin curls. For this style, you must really understand the texture of your hair, as the set must be tight enough to give both body and curl. Back-comb a little at the front if necessary. Courtesy of *Good Housekeeping* magazine. Copyright Hearst Corporation, 1971. Photographer: Francesco Scavullo

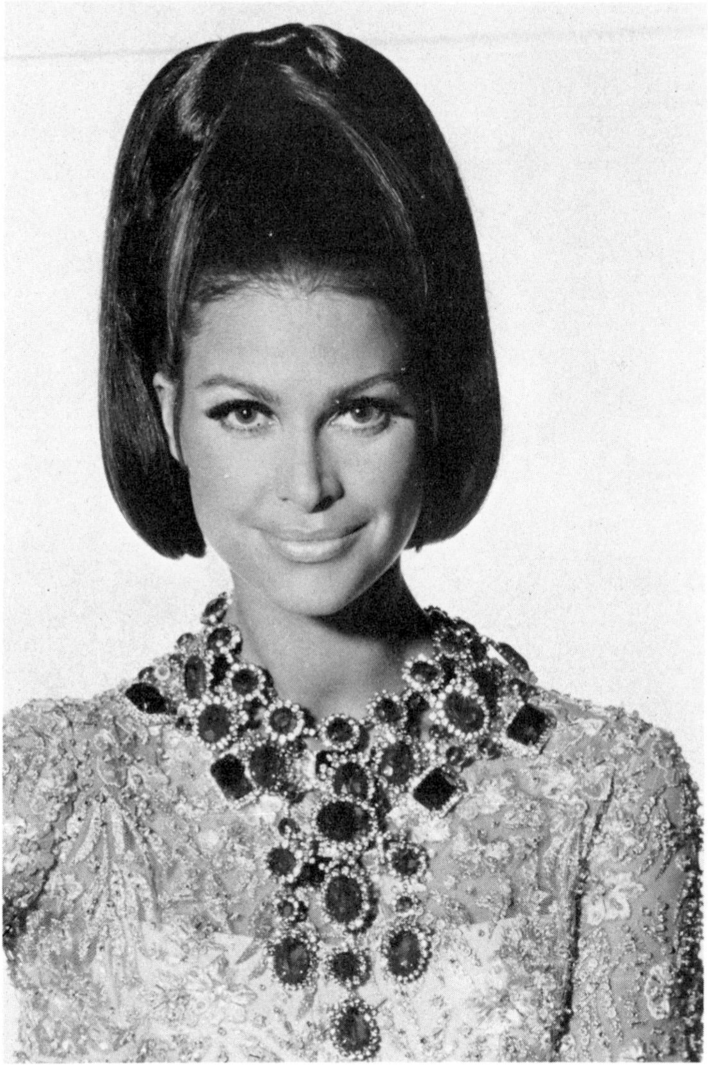

Here is a hair style which represents one of the most important transitional periods of hair. While not a long style, it certainly has a "rich girl look" and the line is still very important today. A short full hairpiece has been incorporated in the back. From *Vogue*, © 1966 by The Condé Nast Publications, Inc.

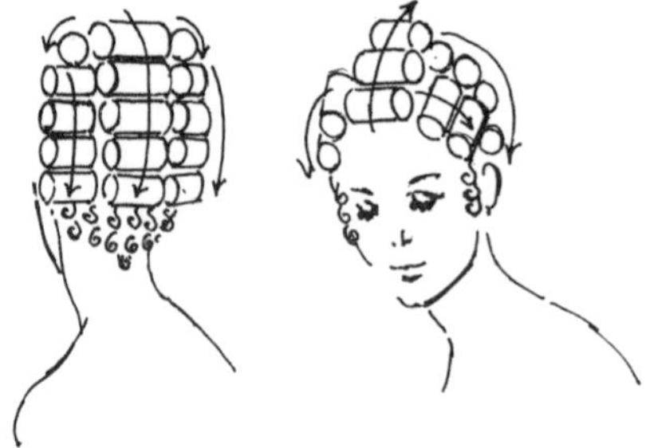

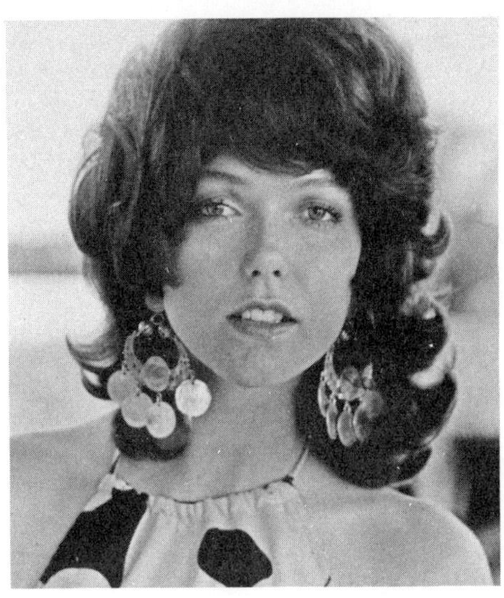

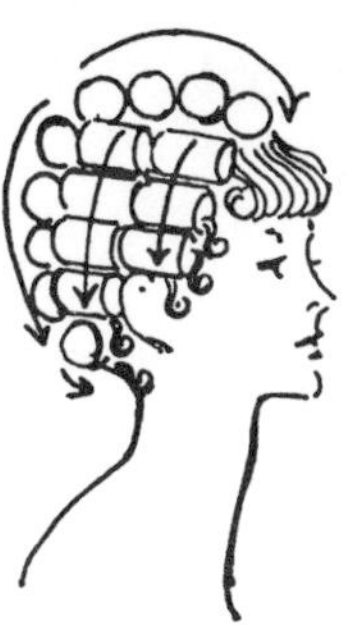

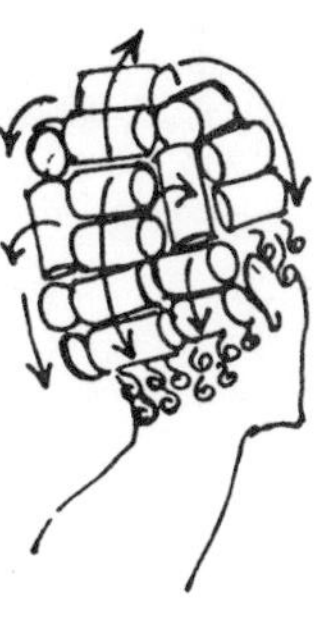

I think this picture proves that blunt-cut layered hair can be very pretty. Rain, wind or snow cannot destroy it if it has a really good cut. If your hair texture is strong enough or you have a slight wave, this can be blown dry but you may also set it. *Woman's Day,* June 1971. Photographer: William Connors

While I have always admired all-one-length hair that moves beautifully, I think this kind of cut that is shorter toward the face is also very flattering. I like its somewhat free, casual feeling and the fact that it's still long enough to move on the head. *Woman's Day,* June 1971. Photographer: William Connors

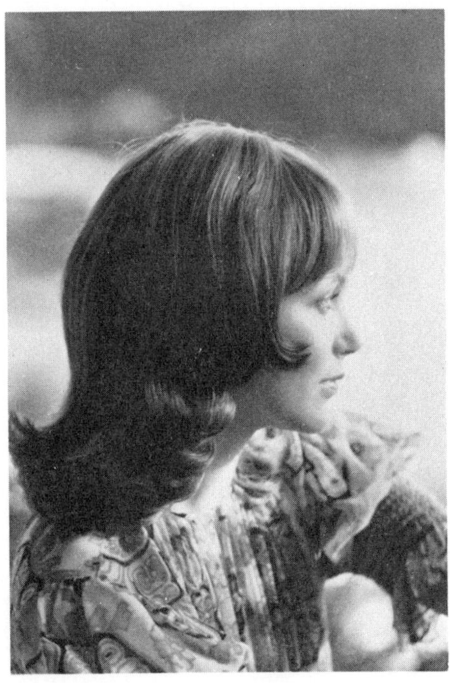

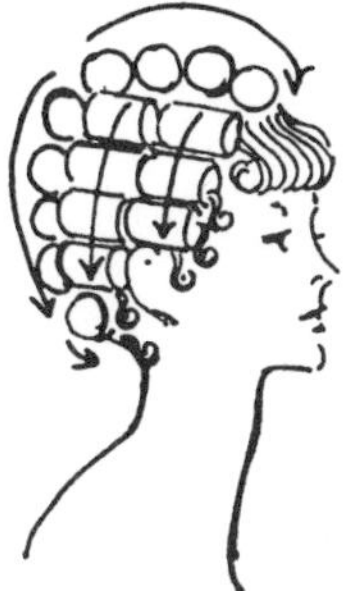

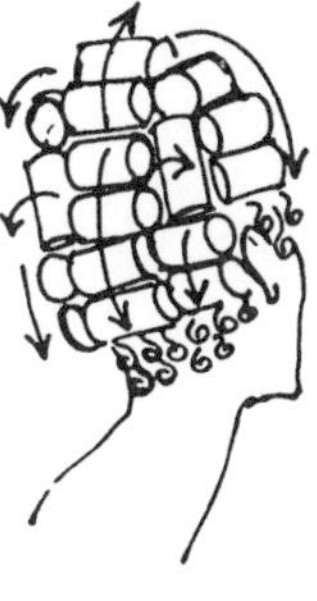

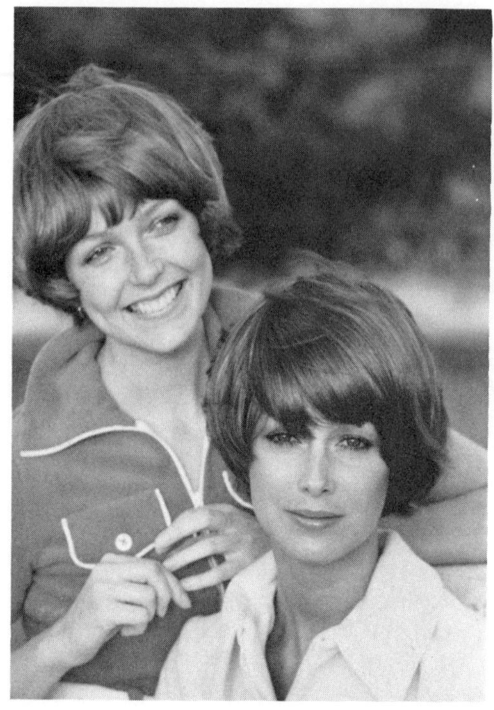

These are two short "little head" wigs of modacrylic fiber. What a pretty way to look during or after a day at the beach. The fact that the cost is under $40 proves how good you can look quite easily today. It's also a practical way to protect your own hair from the sun. *Woman's Day*, June 1971. Photographer: William Connors

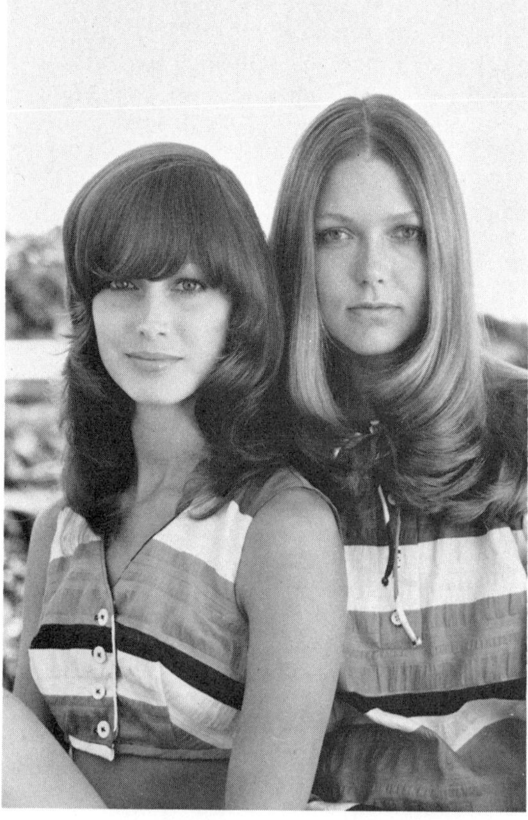

I think this picture says one thing–beautiful, shiny, clean, healthy, luxurious hair. And hair that's superbly cut, kept in great condition and then simply blown dry. *Woman's Day*, June 1971. Photographer: William Connors

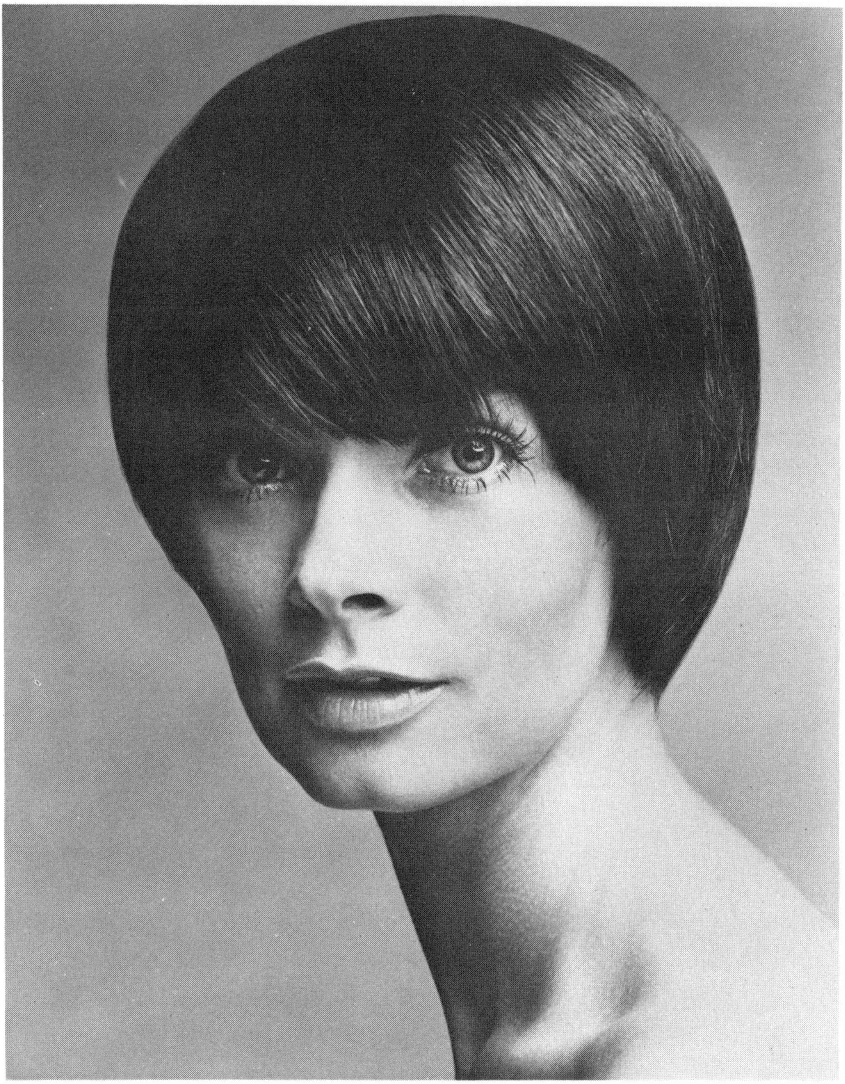

Many women wear a version of this kind of short hairdo. The differences over the years have been the result of the mechanics used to achieve it. It used to be razor cut and thinned, with perhaps only a place set. Today we always scissor-place cut it to keep body in the hair and then blow it dry. Some women like extra lift—a few rollers in the top can achieve this. Photographer: Gordon Munro

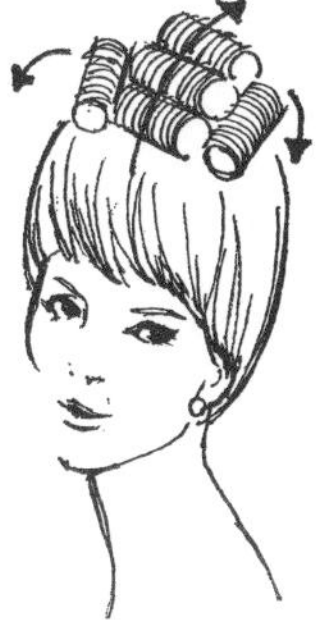

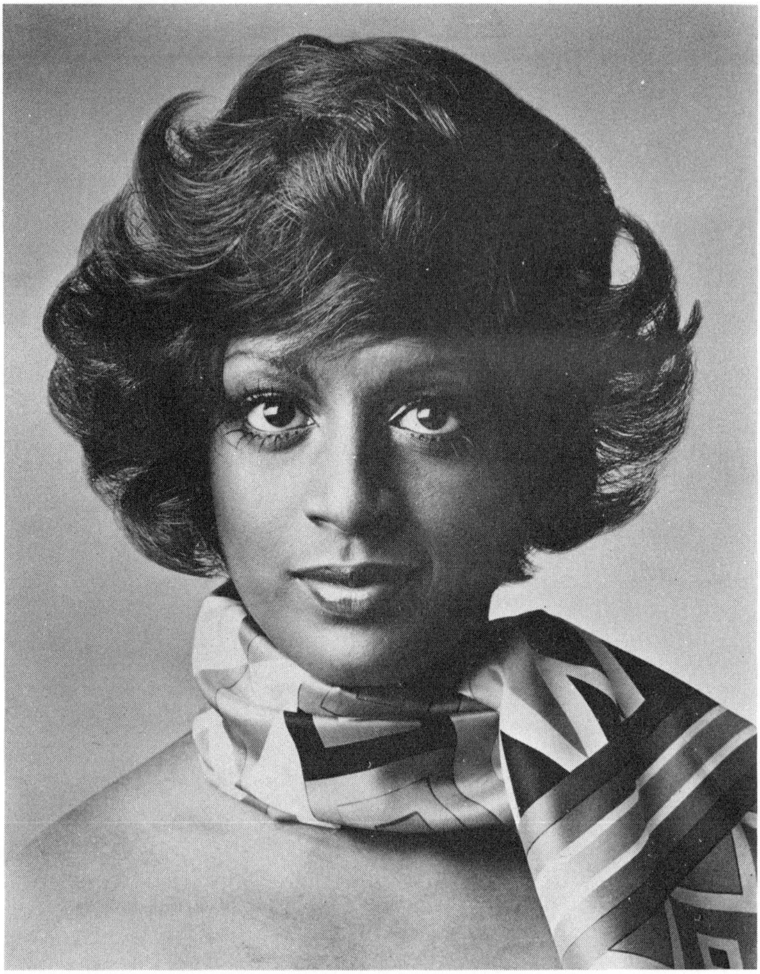

This picture represents a way of wearing hair that I can only refer to as a kind of classic feather cut. Even though the entire head is layered, there is no thinning of the hair and the blunt scissors cut helps control hair that might have too much curl. This can be blown dry if your hair is cut perfectly and has just the right amount of curl. Photographer: Gordon Munro

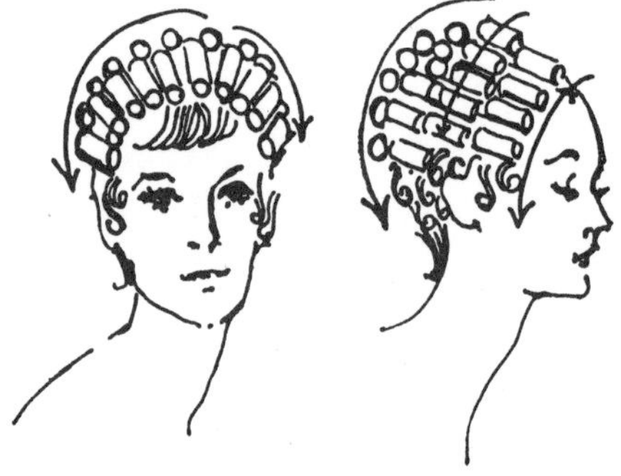

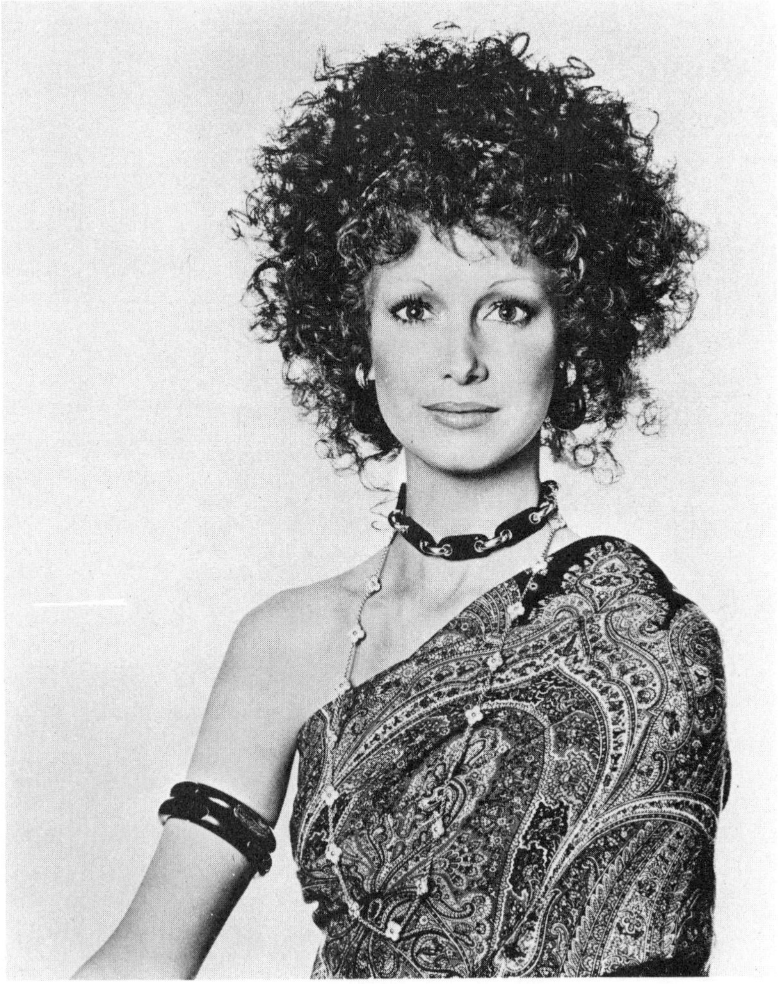

This was a kind of fantasy picture when I did it for *Vogue,* but it has become quite commonplace as a look on the streets. This is the kind of style I would only advise those with authority and security to try, those with that special individual flair for all fashion. From *Vogue,* © 1971 by The Condé Nast Publications, Inc. Photographer: Penn

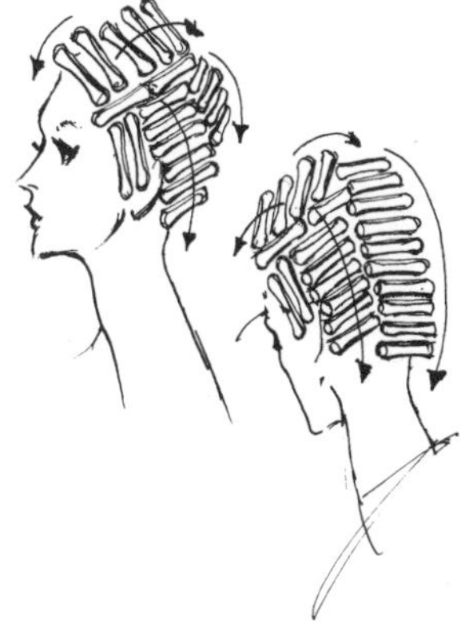

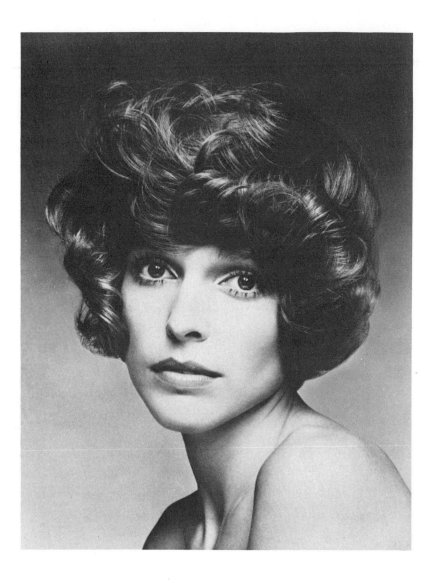

A "cap" of curls for any age from six to sixty and the kind of hairdo that translates well in any color. Please note that the curl is a wide-open "arc," not at all a frizz. This makes it softer and more flattering. (Use 1 to 1½″ rollers.) Photographer: Gordon Munro

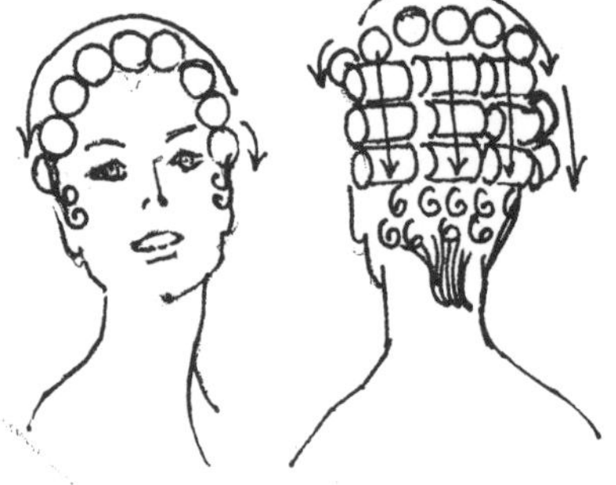

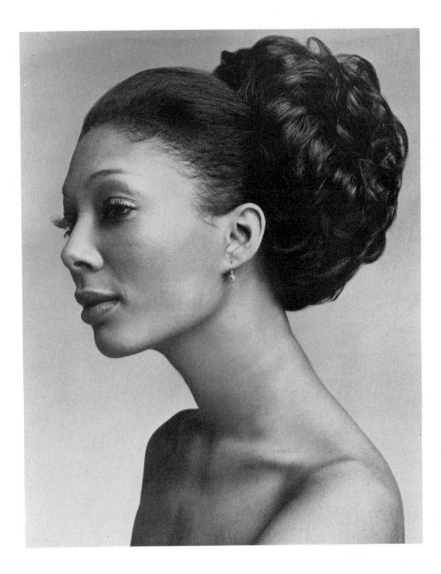

So many black women love to control their hair by pulling it tight to the head and yet sometimes want to expand on the idea for special occasions or special clothes. In this case, the hair is pulled up tightly in a covered elastic and an acrylic fiber wiglet is added for extra line. Photographer: Gordon Munro

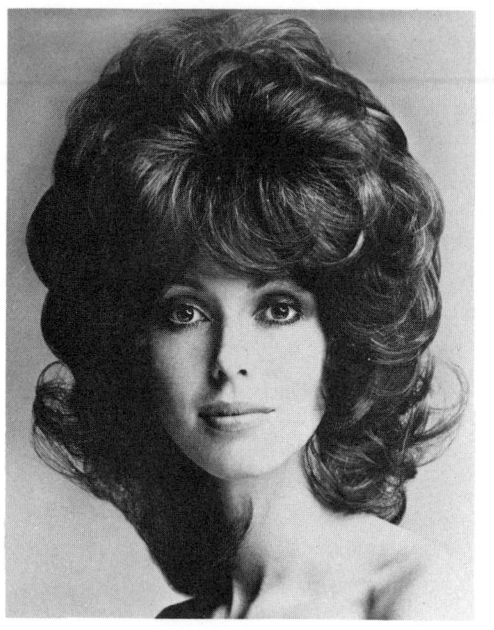

'Use 1½″ rollers.)

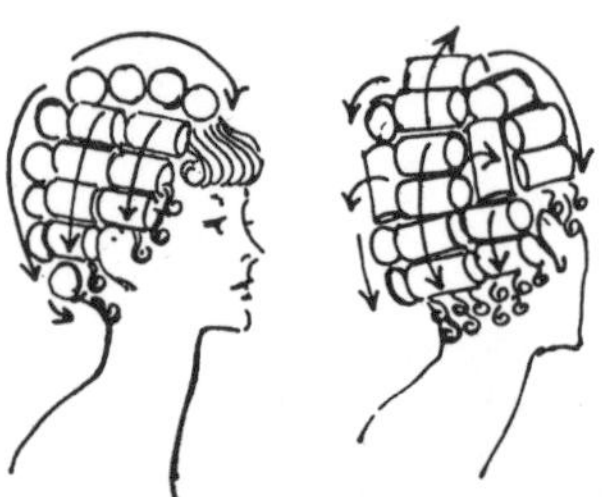

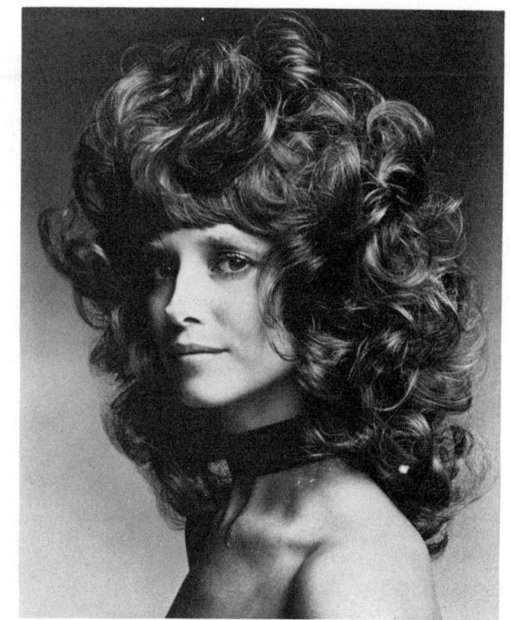

(Use ½″ rollers.)

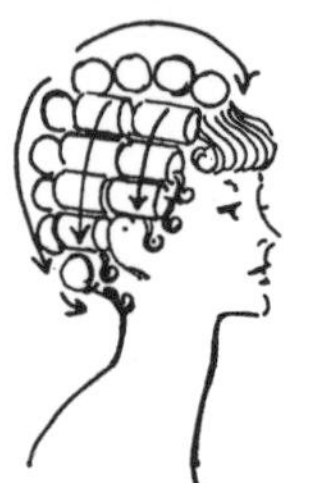

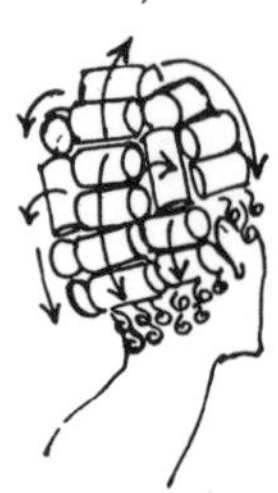

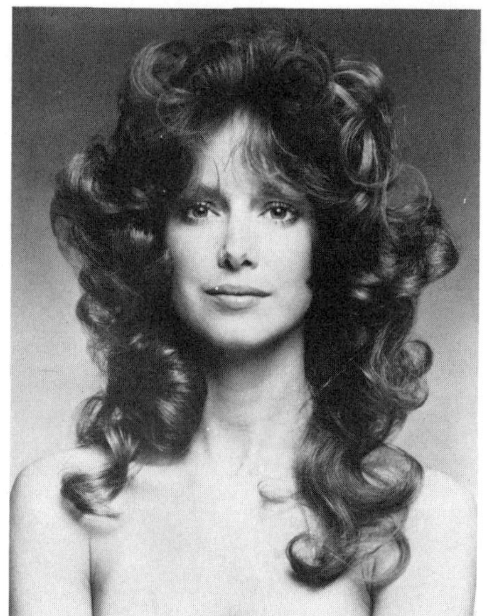

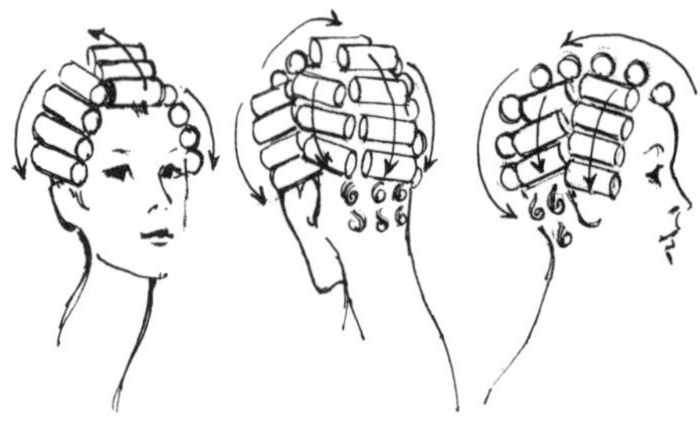

(Use ¾″ rollers.)

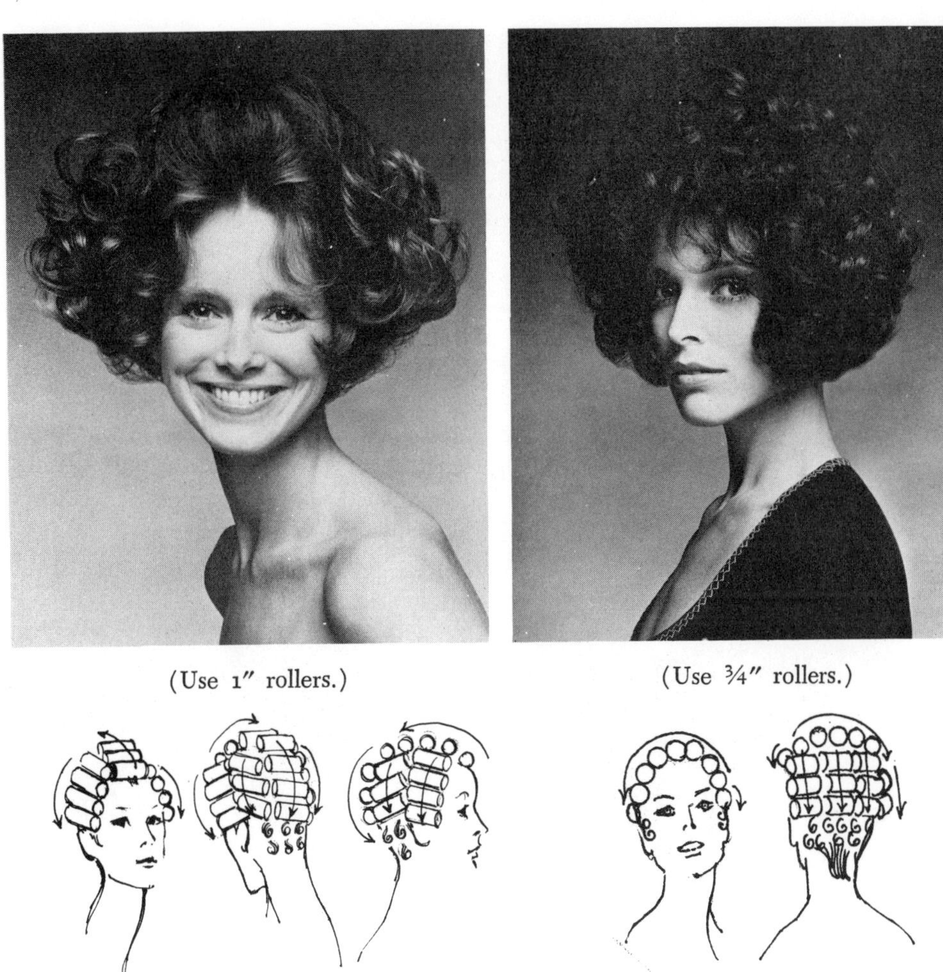

(Use 1″ rollers.)

(Use ¾″ rollers.)

There are women who will never wear the straighter, closer-to-the-head styles that we lean more and more toward because of easy care and maintenance. They want the glamour, the romance and extreme femininity of very full, softly curled, shorter or longer hair. This group represents what I believe are very pretty versions of that kind of hair. Photographer: Gordon Munro

These pictures are proof that most styles are basic in shape and can be varied by size of rollers based on knowledge of your hair texture.

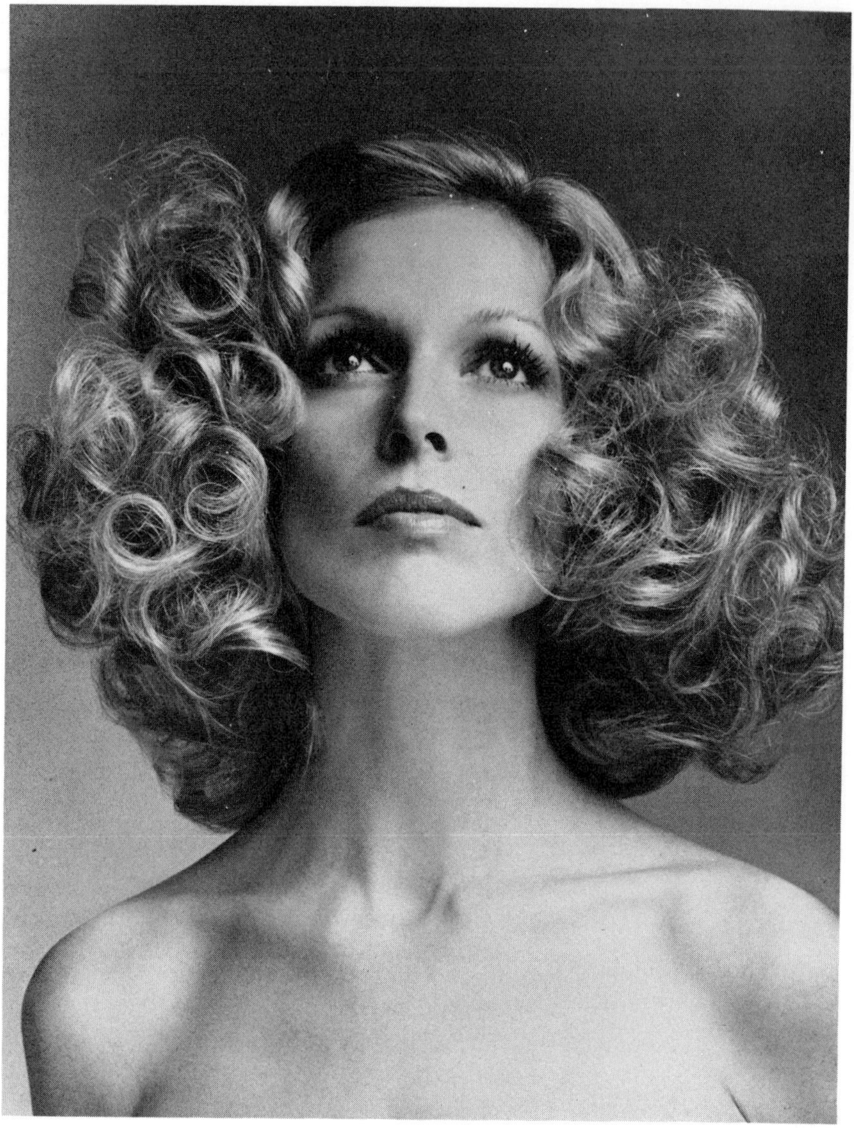

A longer style done mostly on pin curls reminds me of my beginning days, as it has a part as well as the pin-curl setting. Although it is reminiscent, I feel it is very much of the 1970s. Photographer: Gordon Munro

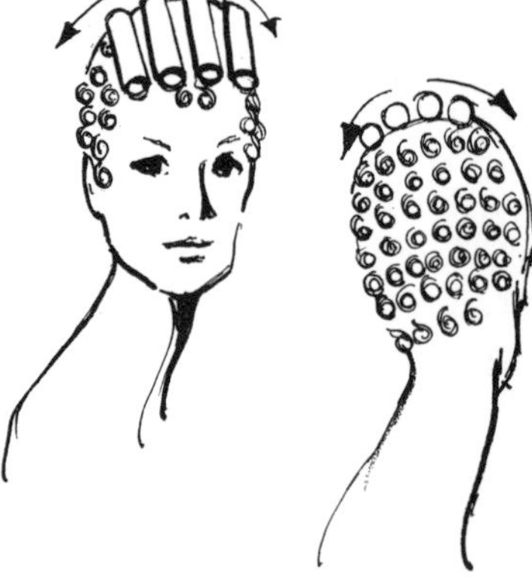

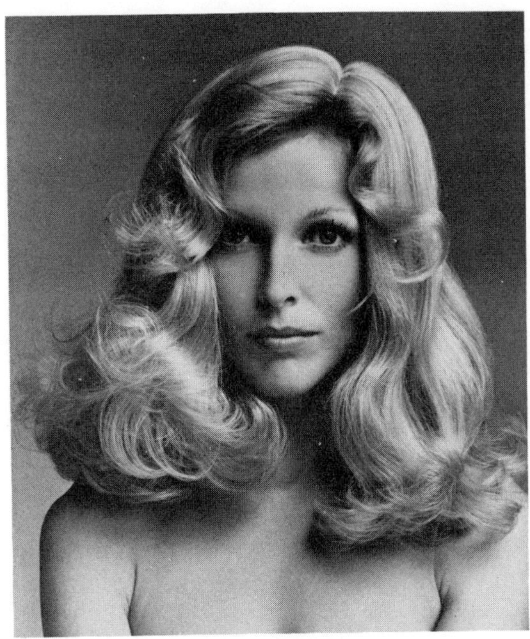

Here is very much longer hair. One style is quite straight with blunt, even ends; the other is wavier and side parted with somewhat more curl at the ends. Most young people really prefer longer hair today and I find these interesting examples as they are both acrylic fiber wigs. This is an aid for the many women who have too fine or too thin hair, or find they have to wash it more than they like. It's truly amazing how much wigs have come along in design and style to look so very real and yet be in the price range of so many people's pocketbooks. Photographer: Gordon Munro

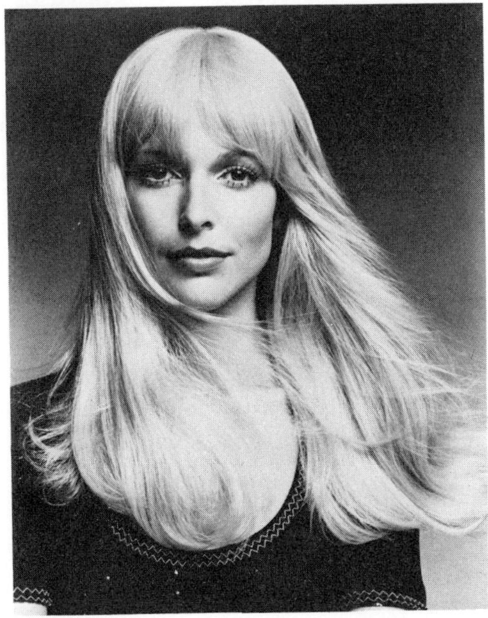

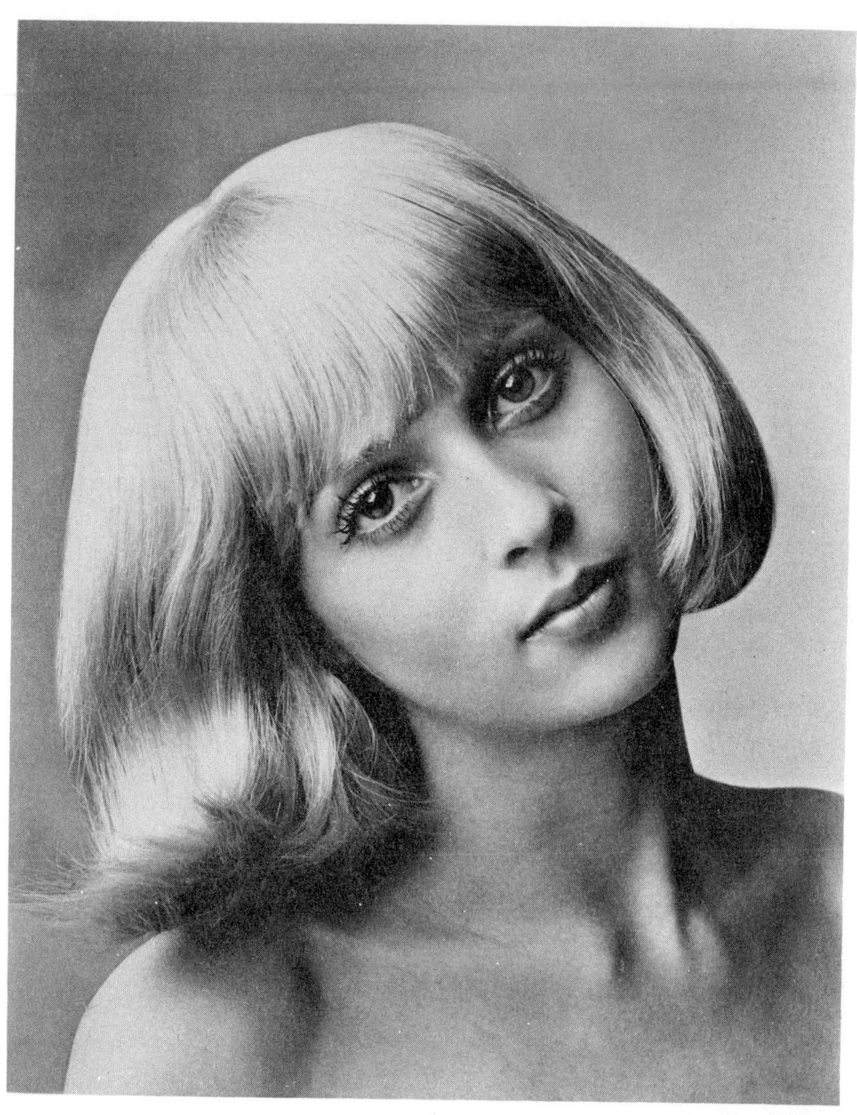

A true classic style—long ago called "Buster Brown" and for many years the favored look of Chanel for her models. Most recently, it's been labeled "Chinese." It is an easy way to cope with one's hair and has changed only because of the mechanical ways in which it's produced. The latest methods and my favorites are blow dry or hot comb. Photographer: Gordon Munro

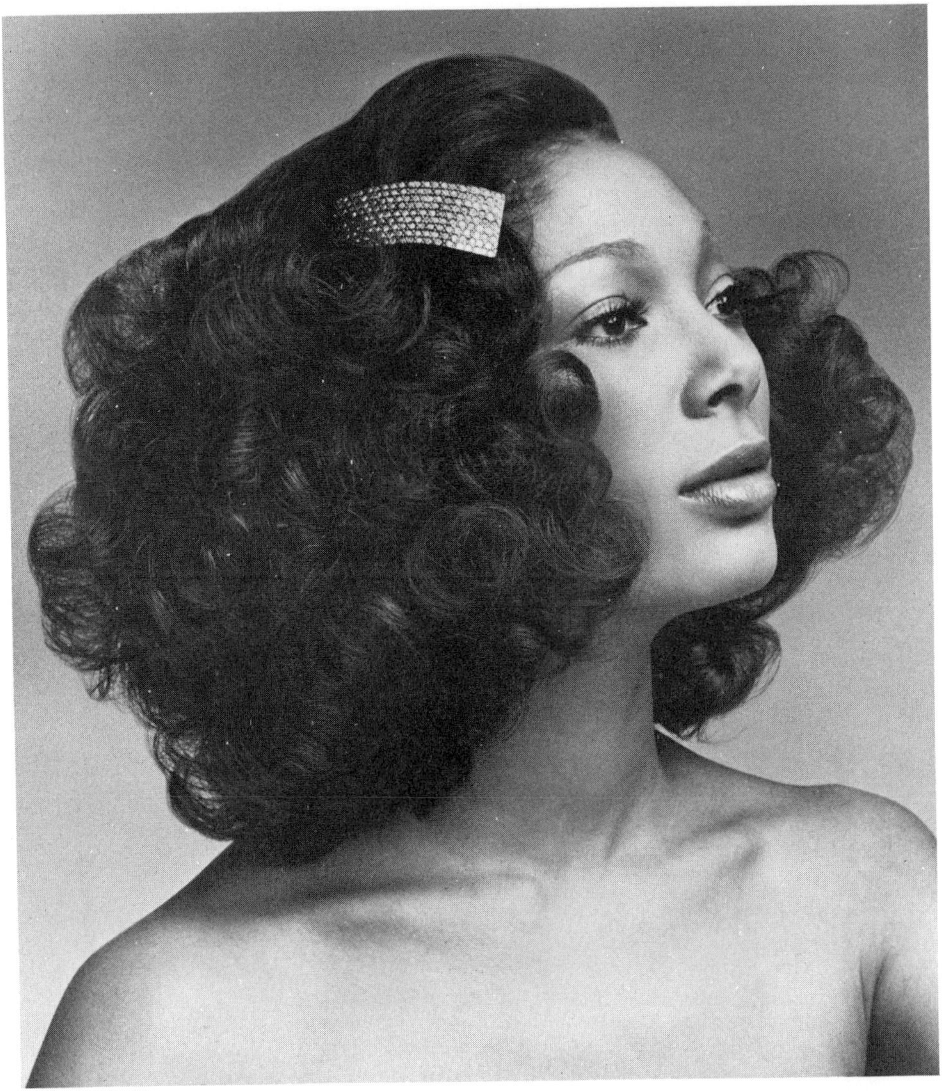

Try this pretty way to cope with naturally very curly hair. It's basically a curly style and yet has definite line because of a smooth top and perhaps a side part. It can be done with a pin-curl or roller setting, depending on which works better for your hair.
Photographer: Gordon Munro

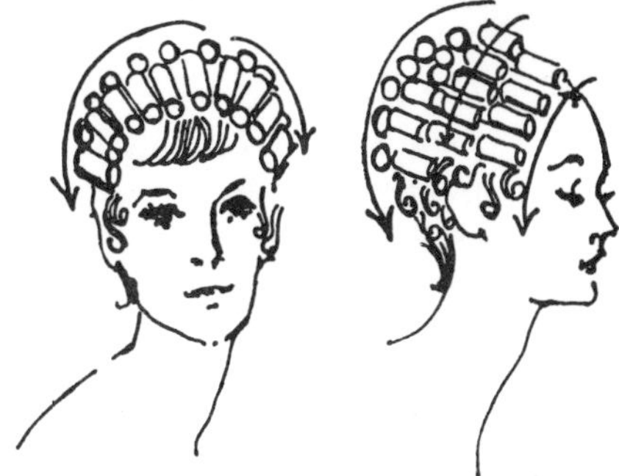

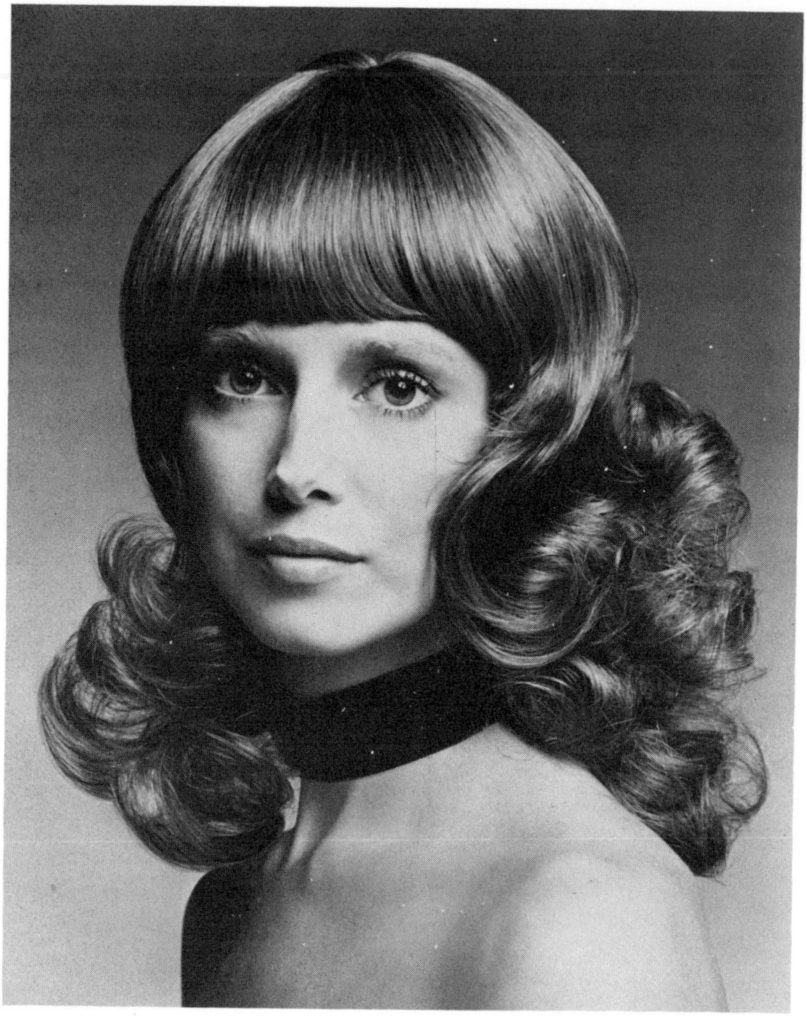

For growing-out layered hair, when a smoother look is desired and yet one does not want to cut off the length while the hair evens out, this style is perfect. I think it has great appeal and is a good solution for a vexing problem especially after so many Shag haircuts. Use large (2″) rollers at the top and crown and switch to smaller rollers (¾″) at the sides and bottom. Photographer: Gordon Munro

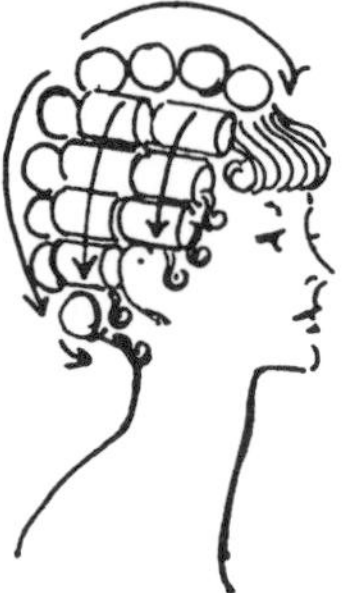

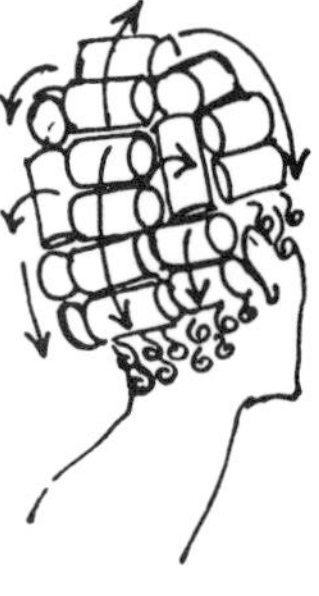

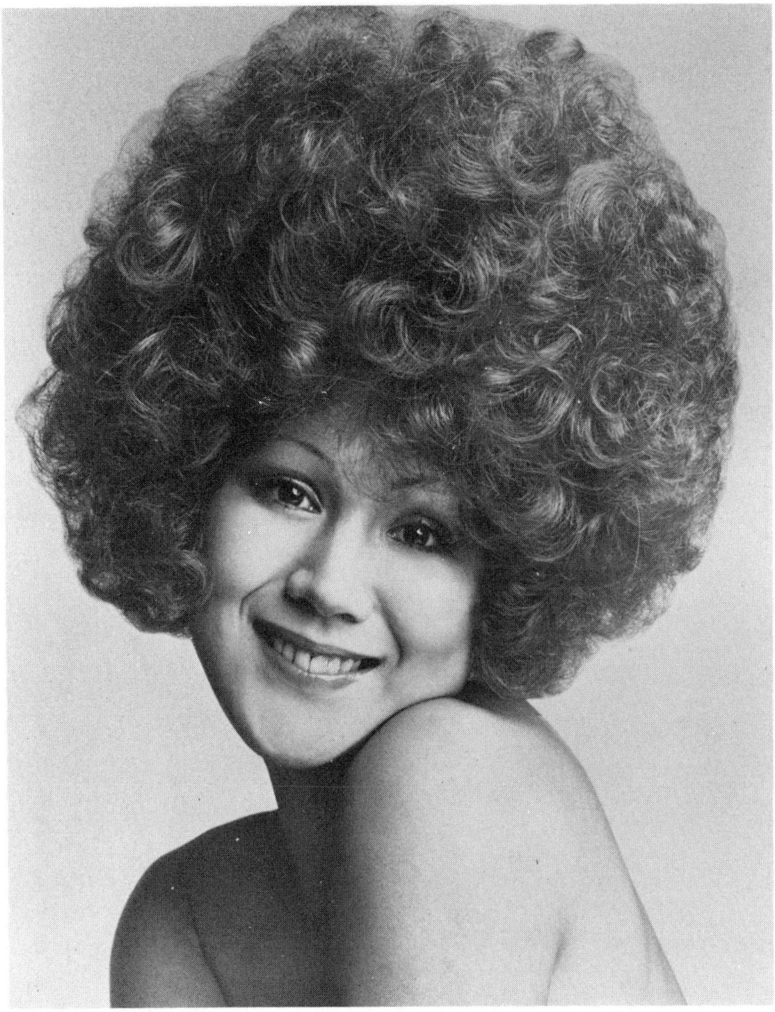

It's marvelous today to think that curly hair is no longer a curse. Here is medium-short hair almost allowed to do its own thing and cut well enough that even when the hair does "revert," it will have a good shape. Photographer: Gordon Munro

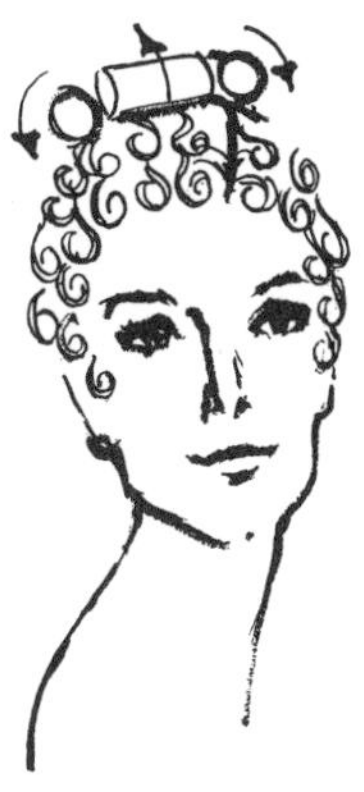

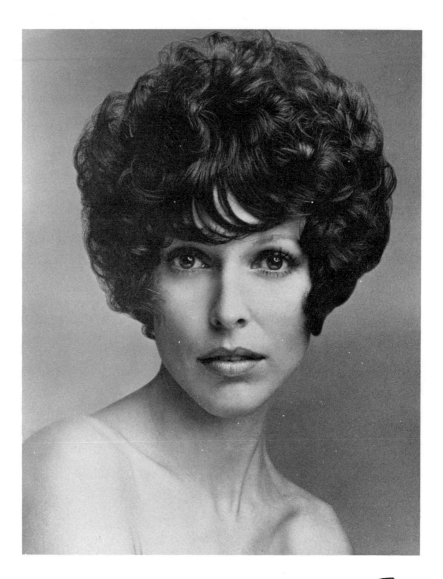

This is about the shortest I like to see curly hair as I don't like cropped hair when it's extremely curly. If it's too short you get a frizz instead of the full turn of a curl. Photographer: Gordon Munro

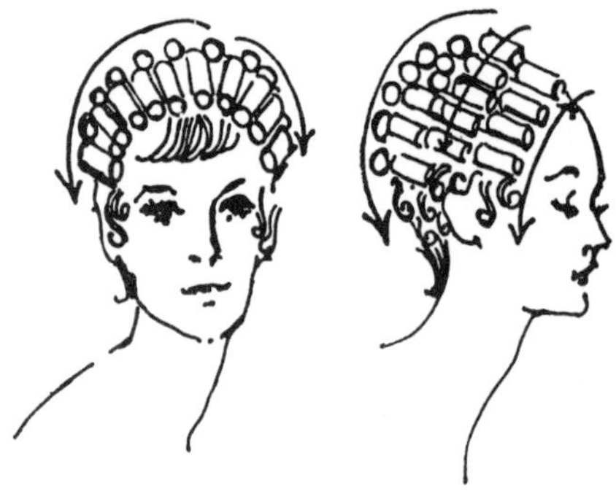

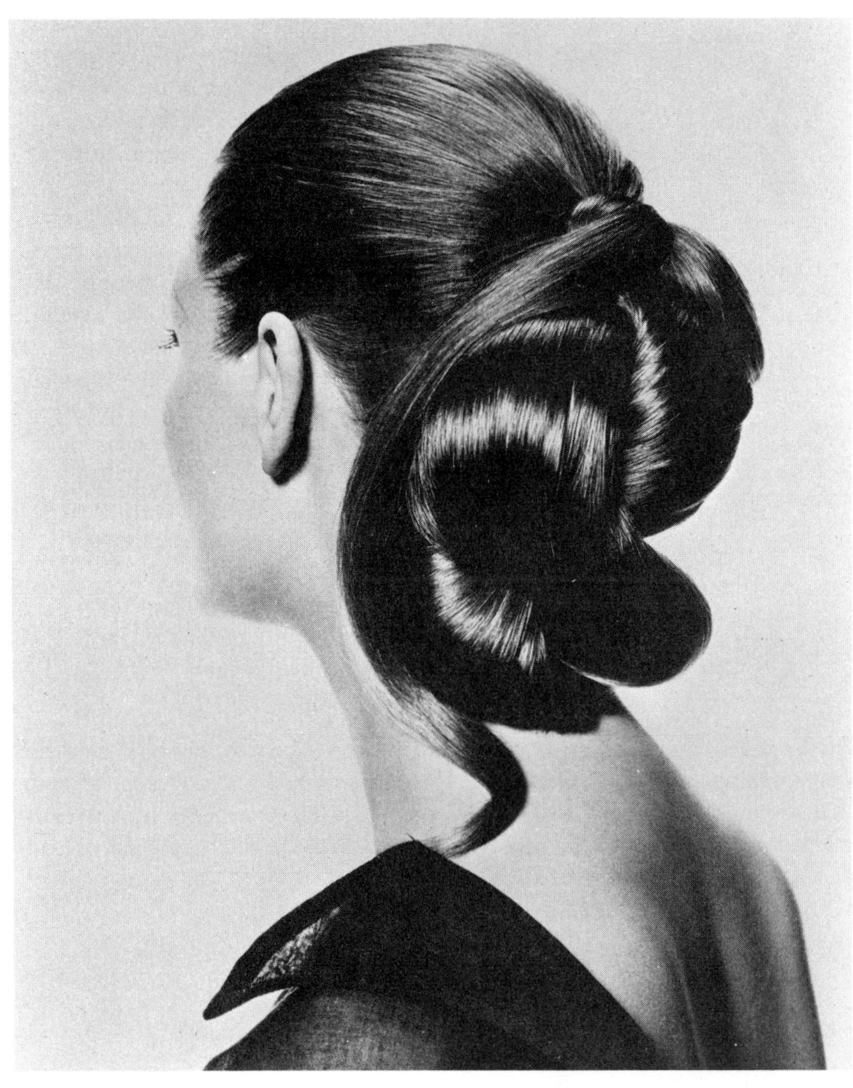

A picture that says more about luxurious hair than any words ever could. Use your own long hair if you have it by pulling it back into a covered elastic, then twisting the end until it loops back up on itself. Or incorporate a synthetic switch if you like. This is a take-off on a classic Figure 8. From *Vogue*, © 1965 by The Condé Nast Publications, Inc. Photographer: Penn

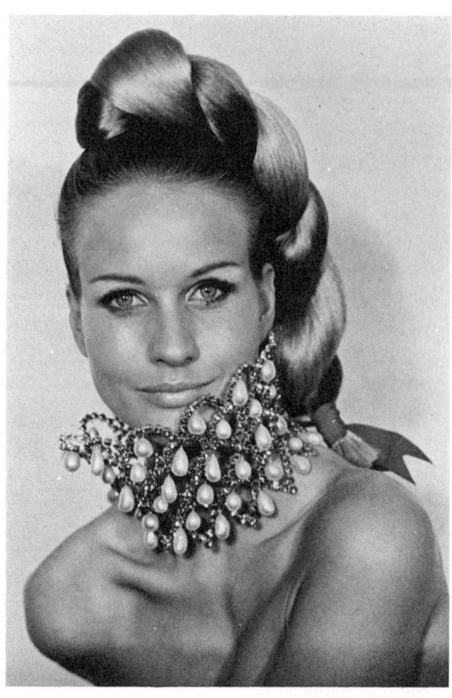

One of the simplest ways to cope with your hair on a vacation or in the tropics or when you don't have time to go to the hairdresser. So often, in those circumstances, women try to make their hair do things it just won't do because of the humidity or the salt air. Each of you should have a trick or two, like this one, so you don't have to fuss with your hair when you're having fun. This is hair simply pulled back, then a synthetic braided switch added. From *Vogue*, © 1968 by The Condé Nast Publications, Inc. Photographer: Franco Rubartelli

This setting was two days old when the picture was made, because we were photographing a beach beauty story. The hair was brushed and combed with whatever curl it still had, and a bandeau with some attached synthetic curls was tied around like a Juliet cap. I think I produced a pretty, ingenuous and romantic look for a quickie hairdo. *Woman's Day,* June 1971. Photographer: William Connors

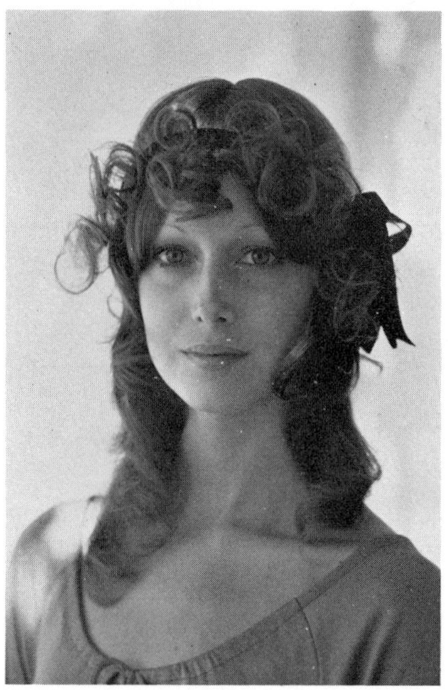

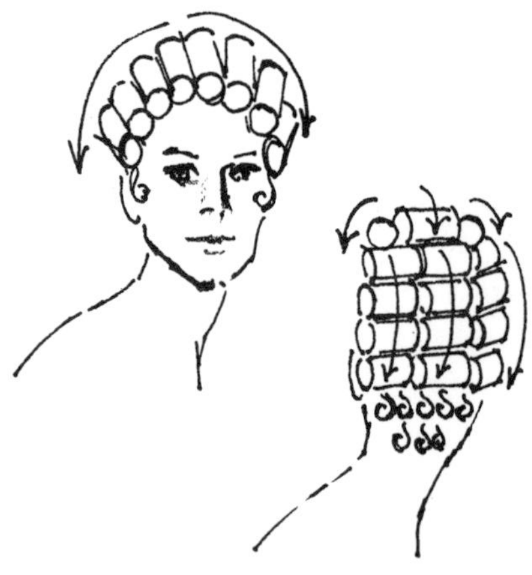

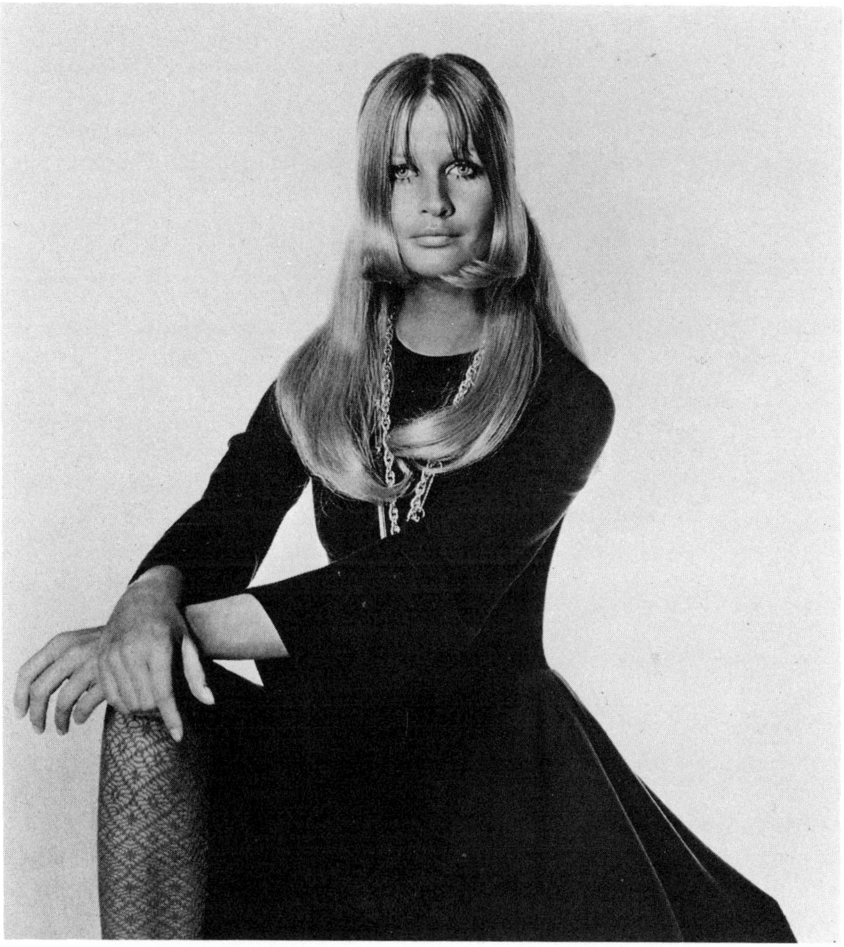

A lot of girls wear their hair this way if they want it long, because there's a second layer around the face for a softer effect. Many girls have become tired of just plain long hair, but they don't want to cut it off. The double layer of hair—or two-layer hair—gives them definition but still long hair. Most all the girls I know who wear this kind of hair do not set it, but if you want to set it you can. But use very large (2″) rollers so that the hair is just bent and not really curled. From *Vogue*, © 1968 by The Condé Nast Publications, Inc.

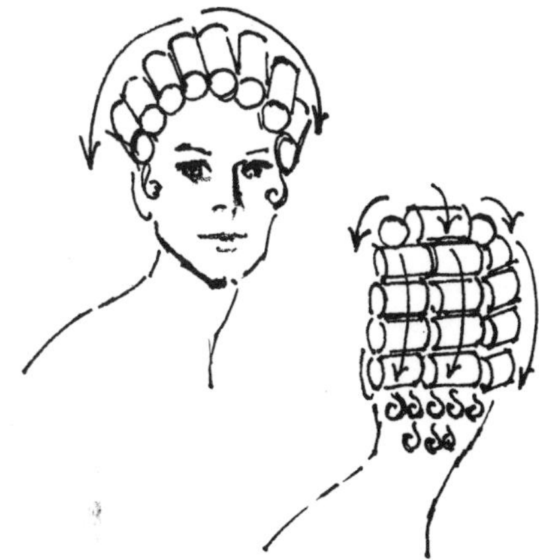

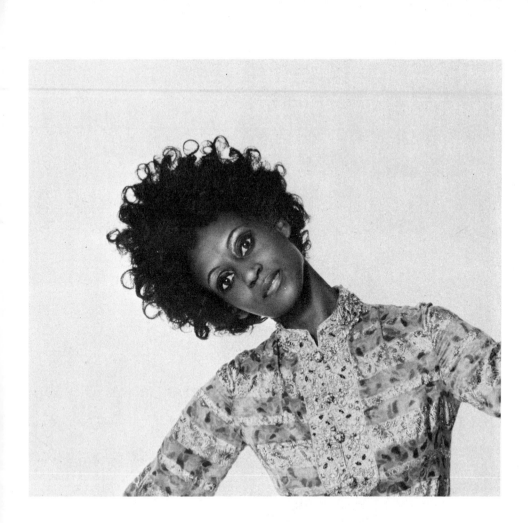

Here's a so-called "natural" shape, but without the almost topiary quality that many women prefer. It's a bit more loosely curled and is finished with curly ends that you can see light through them. It can be a nice change. If your hair is curly enough you could set this on pin curls, but permanent-wave rods will give you a longer lasting set. From *Vogue*, © 1969 by The Condé Nast Publications, Inc.

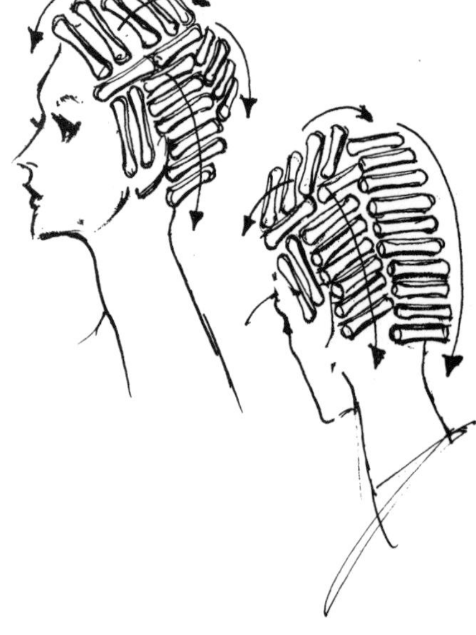

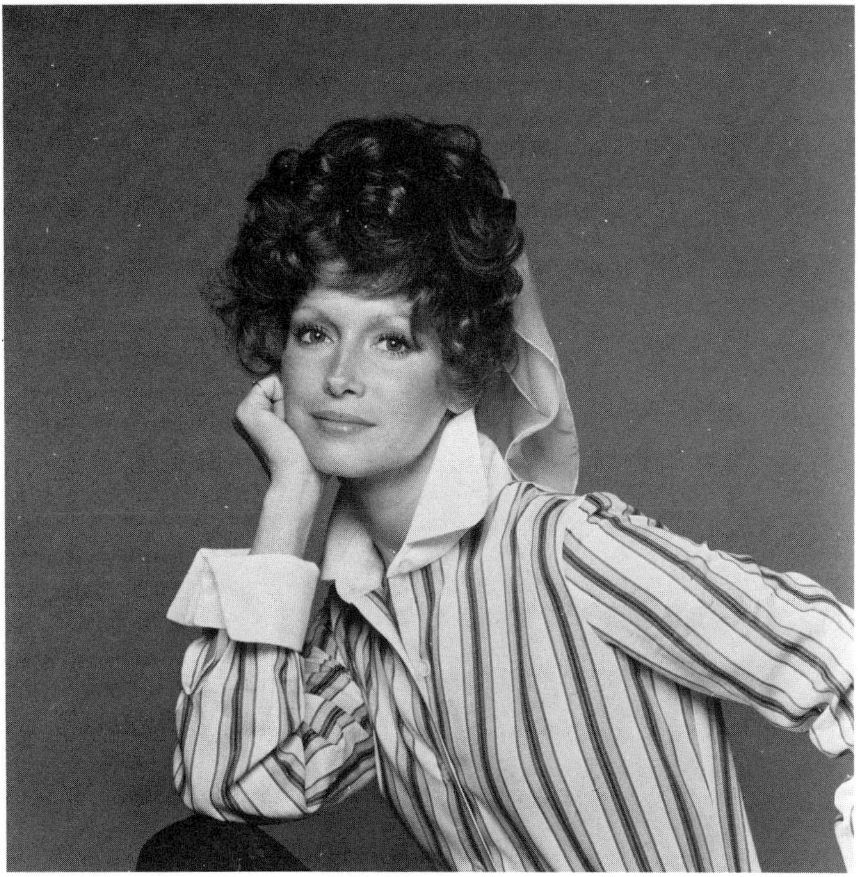

I did this hair recently when the "return of the '40s" first hit the scene. It's fascinating to me that now, in the '70s, this look has returned. This hair style has the faintest touch of nostalgia, but it is contemporary. The real difference comes from the improvements in techniques and materials we have to work with today. Courtesy of *Good Housekeeping* magazine. Copyright Hearst Corporation, 1971.

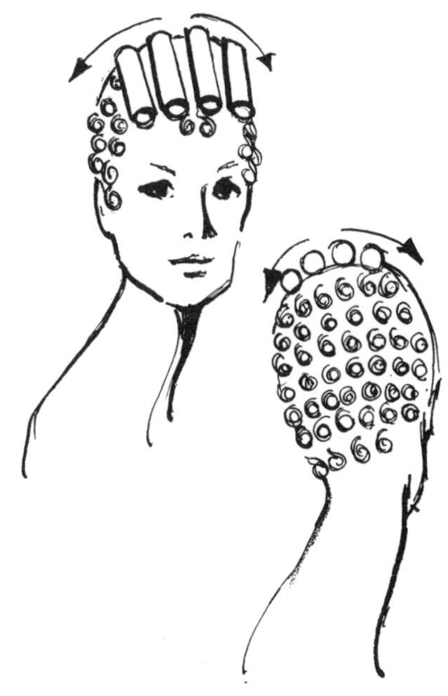